A Week of Switching, Shifting, and Stretching

How to Make My Thinking More Flexible

Lauren H. Kerstein, LCSW

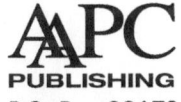

AAPC
PUBLISHING
P.O. Box 23173
Shawnee Mission, Kansas 66283-0173
www.aapcpublishing.net

AAPC PUBLISHING

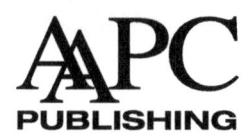

©2014 AAPC Publishing
P.O. Box 23173
Shawnee Mission, Kansas 66283-0173
www.aapcpublishing.net

All rights reserved. No part of the material protected by this copyright notice may be reproduced or used in any form or by any means, electronic or mechanical, including photocopying, recording, or by any information storage and retrieval system, without the prior written permission of the copyright owner.

Publisher's Cataloging-in-Publication

Kerstein, Lauren H.

A week of switching, shifting, and stretching : how to make my thinking more flexible / Lauren H. Kerstein. -- Shawnee Mission, Kan. : AAPC Publishing, c2014.

p. ; cm.

ISBN: 978-1-937473-89-1
LCCN: 2013952005

Includes bibliographical references.

Summary: An illustrated children's book teaching children the importance of being flexible in daily life. The first part is for children, followed by a section for parents and professionals containing activities designed to support and generalize the infor mation.--Publisher.

1. Children with autism spectrum disorders --Behavior modification. 2. Autistic children --Behavior modification. 3. Problem solving in children. 4. Stress management for children. 5. Adaptability (Psychology) in children. 6. Adjustment (Psychology) in child ren. 7. [Autism --Life skills guides. 8. Problem solving. 9. Stress management. 10. Interpersonal relations. 11. Social skills.] I. Title.

RJ506.A9 K47 2014
618.92/85882--dc23   1310

This book is designed in Calibri.

Illustrations ©iClipart.com

Printed in the United States of America.

Dedication

This book is dedicated to my daughters, who are beautiful inside and out. Being a mother for the past decade has been the greatest joy and the greatest challenge of my life thus far. Sarah Hailey and Danielle Emily, you have given me a crash course in becoming more flexible so that I might provide a better model. I hope that you are able to be true to yourselves, celebrate your accomplishments, learn from your challenges, and stretch your minds as far as you can.

Josh, I don't know where I'd be without you by my side on this crazy journey. Our daughters are so lucky to have you as their daddy. I am so lucky to have your support and encouragement. I love you.

Acknowledgments

This book would not have been possible without the support of a lot of people.

First, Drs. Nancy Cason and Claire Dumke: Thank you for reading this manuscript in its rawest form in Florida at the Autism Society of America Conference many years ago. We were sitting in a restaurant eating lunch when you gave me your encouragement to go forward with this manuscript. You are truly outstanding clinicians. Thank you for being a part of my life!

Mom: Each day, I am grateful to be your daughter. You have taught me so much about being flexible, about determination, courage, being meticulous, and most important, what it feels like to be loved unconditionally. Thank you.

Dad: You are missed every day. "Because I knew you, I have been changed for good." (*Wicked*)

Amy: Thank you for supporting me and always being there for me.

Kirsten: You are quite possibly the best editor in the world. My books are so much stronger as a result of your wisdom. I truly enjoy every minute of working with you. Thank you.

Vivian: Thank you for your patience, hard work, and incredible talent. Your illustrations clearly capture the essence of this book.

Additional thanks to ALL of the wonderful staff at AAPC, including Keith and Ginny.

Thank you to all of my family and friends who stand behind me with "pom poms" cheering me on. I am so incredibly lucky to have such people in my life. Heather (my dear friend and secret editor) – your wisdom runs deeper than you'll ever know. Ester – there are no words to capture the depth of our friendship. Cheryl, Jamie, Megan, David, Wendy, Ryan, Jenna, Suzi, Stanley, Mimi, Aunt Ellen, and Uncle Jon – I don't know where I'd be without your friendship, love, and support.

To all of the children, adolescents, adults, and families who have given me the honor of walking beside you on your journeys: You inspire me more than I could begin to describe. I hope you believe in yourselves and your ability to grow as much as I believe in you.

– L.H.K.

Hi! My name is Jason and I have a story to tell about my brain.

I have a terrific brain filled with lots of stuff. I even have great ideas.

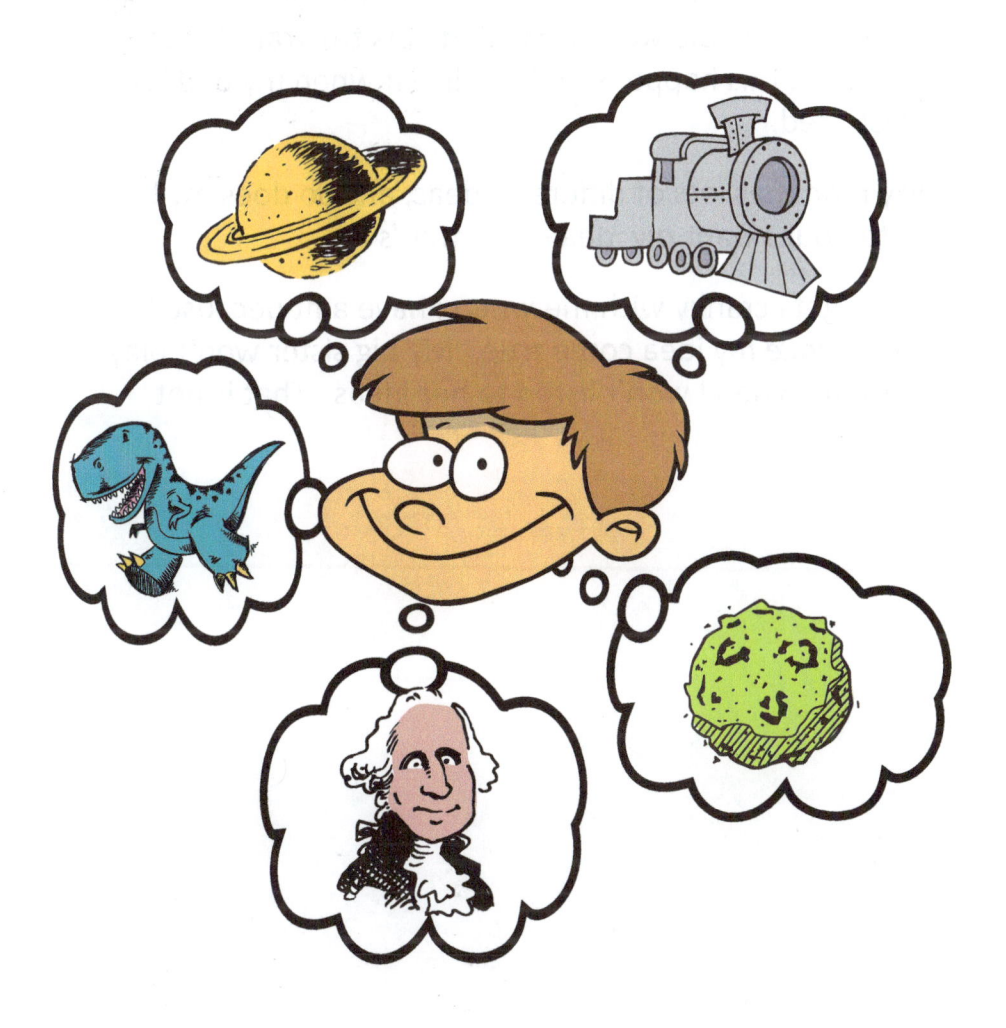

When I get an idea in my head, I want to stick to it. I don't want to change; I don't want to think about other possibilities. I want *my* idea – and that's it!

My dad tells me to think "big." He says there are other ideas that might be great. But I think my idea is the only idea in the whole world. My dad gets frustrated with me when this happens. I don't like it when my dad is frustrated.

My mom has lots of different ideas, and so does my big sister, but I want *my* idea – and that's it.

Mom gets cranky with me when I have a fit because I can't *make* my idea come true. My big sister won't play with me when I won't listen to her ideas. That is not fun!

How to Make My Thinking More Flexible

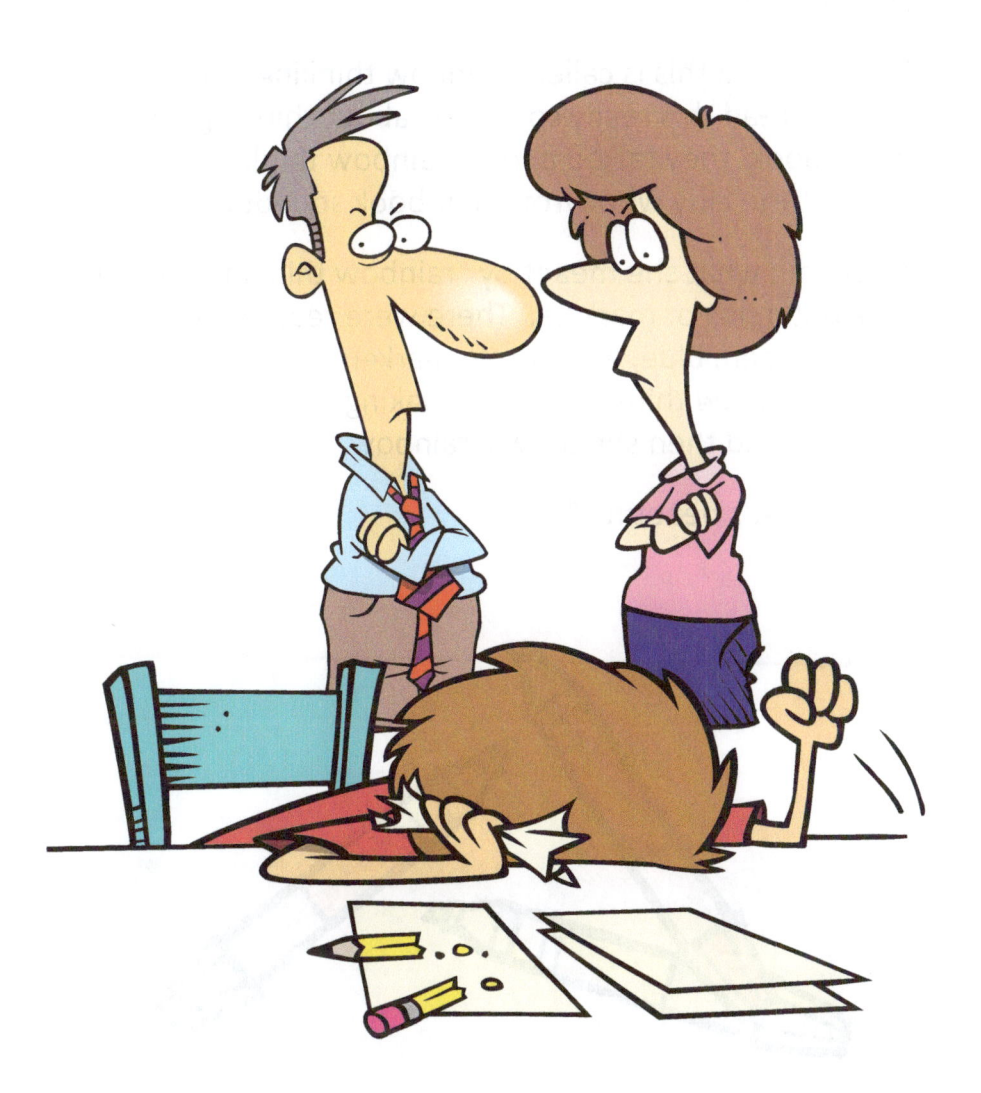

But the other day I learned something interesting.

Ideas can change. They can stretch and shift. They can even switch.

My mom said this is called "rainbow thinking." She said she read this really cool book about thinking BIG.* In the book, they talked about "rainbow thinking." I thought the lady who wrote that book sounded cool.

To explain what she meant by "rainbow thinking," Mom took out a box of markers. There were red, orange, yellow, green, blue, and purple markers. She said that using "rainbow thinking" is like making a rainbow out of markers, and then she drew a rainbow.

"Wow, that's beautiful."

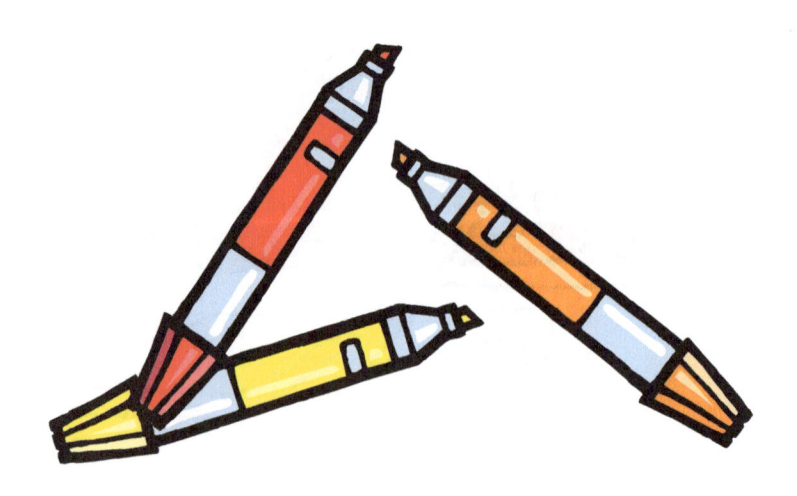

* Collucci, A. (2011). *Big picture thinking: Using central coherence theory to support social skills.* Shawnee Mission, KS: AAPC Publishing.

How to Make My Thinking More Flexible

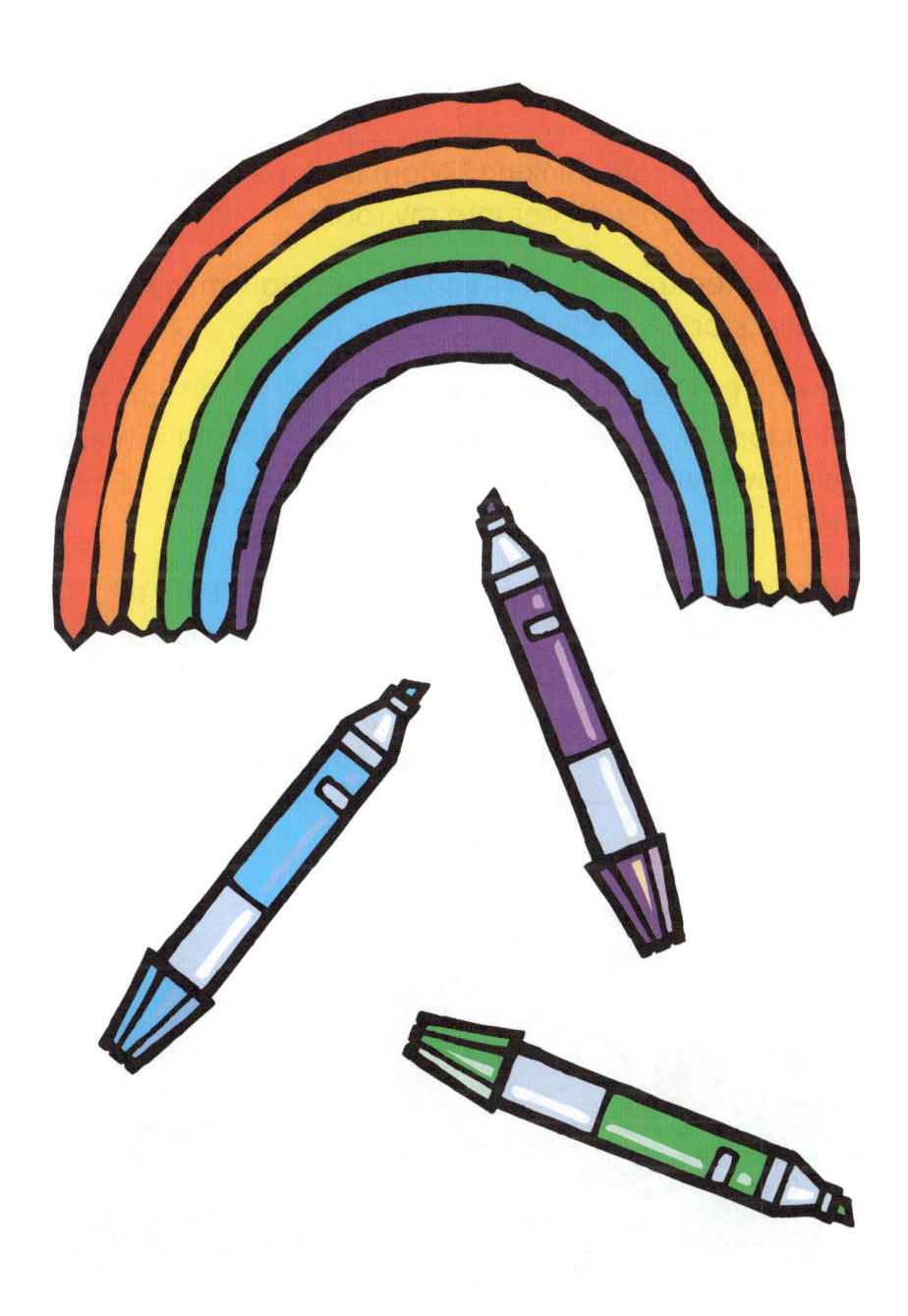

"Rainbow thinking helps us stretch our minds really far. Sometimes you get stuck because you are thinking 'black' or 'white.' Black-and-white thinking isn't nearly as fun as rainbow thinking," Mom told me, and then she asked me to go with her into my room.

She pointed to all my cars and asked, "How many cars are black or white?"

Hmm ... I wondered, looking at the huge pile of cars on the floor. One, two ... I suddenly realized that I actually only have two cars that are black or white, and told my mom.

"That's right, Jason," Mom agreed. "The rest are all the different colors of the rainbow, and that makes them more fun! In fact, if you try to switch, shift, and stretch your thoughts, you might find something great; magnificent; fantastic! You might find a rainbow!"

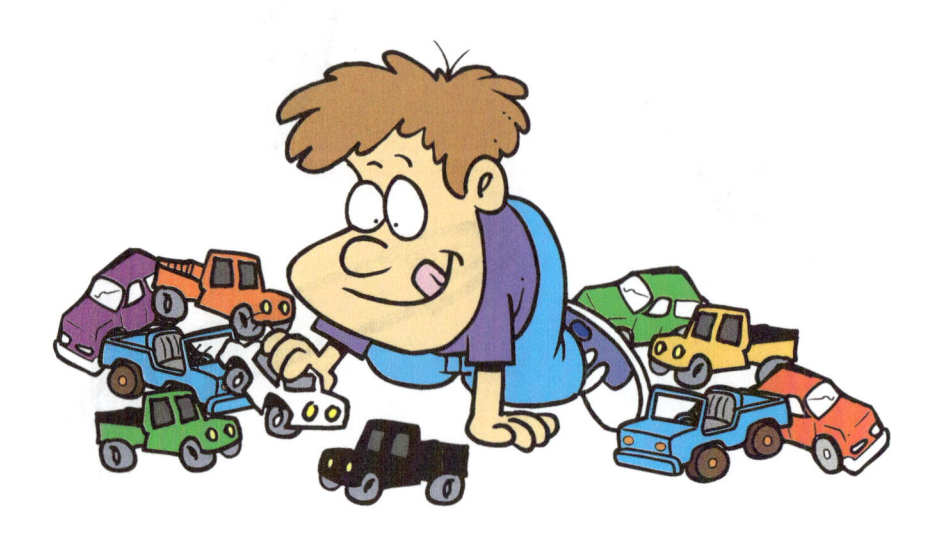

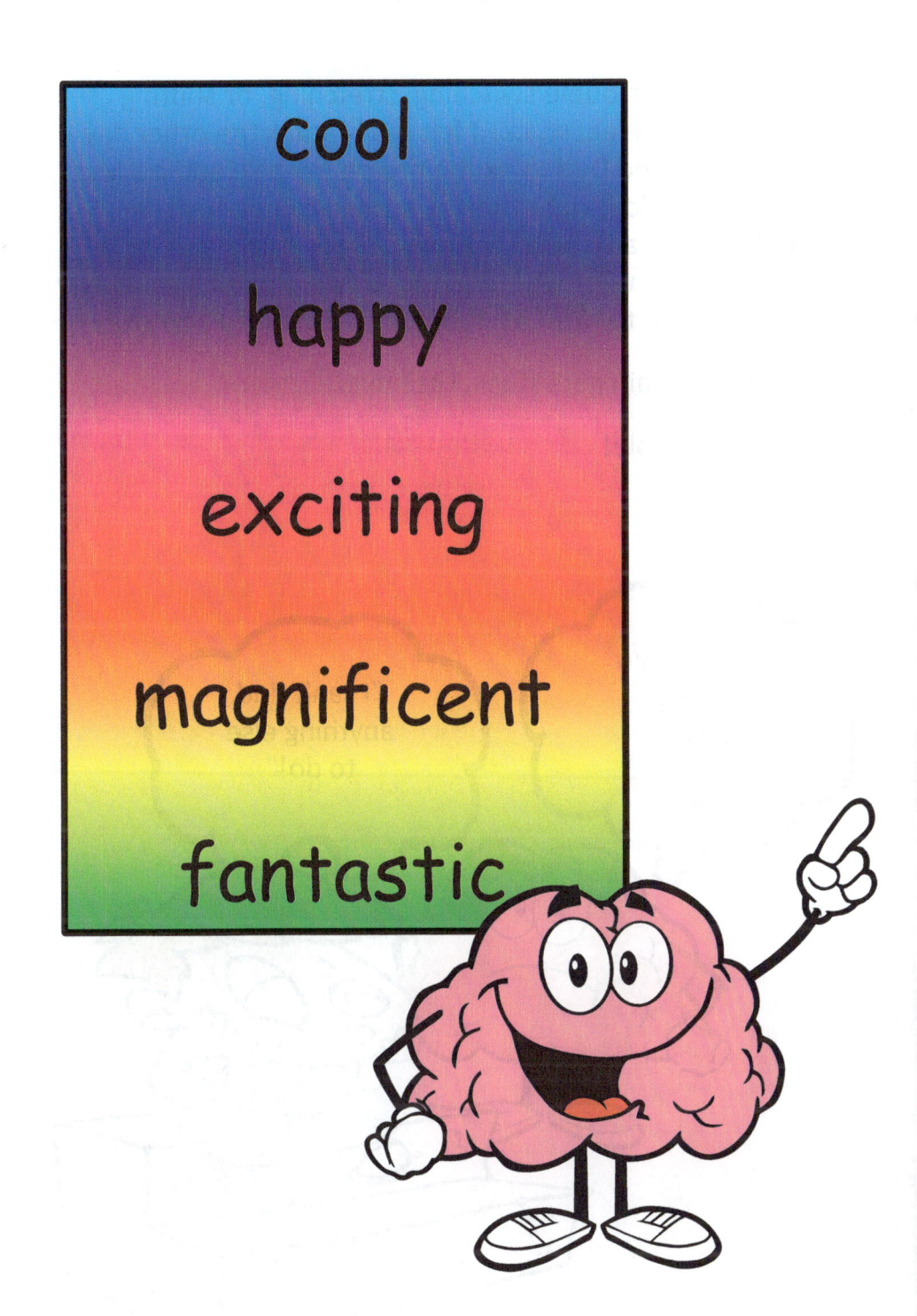

How to Make My Thinking More Flexible

cool

happy

exciting

magnificent

fantastic

A Week of Switching, Shifting, and Stretching

When I have trouble switching, stretching, or shifting my thinking, I feel stuck. I felt really stuck the other day when I wanted Dad to fix the tire on my bike and he was too busy to do it right then. I wanted to ride my bike. I couldn't find anything else to do. I got stuck imagining riding my shiny, green bike. I wouldn't do anything else. I just wanted to ride. I felt bored and grumpy and *stuck*.

When my brain gets stuck, I get mad!

I feel miserable!

I need help!

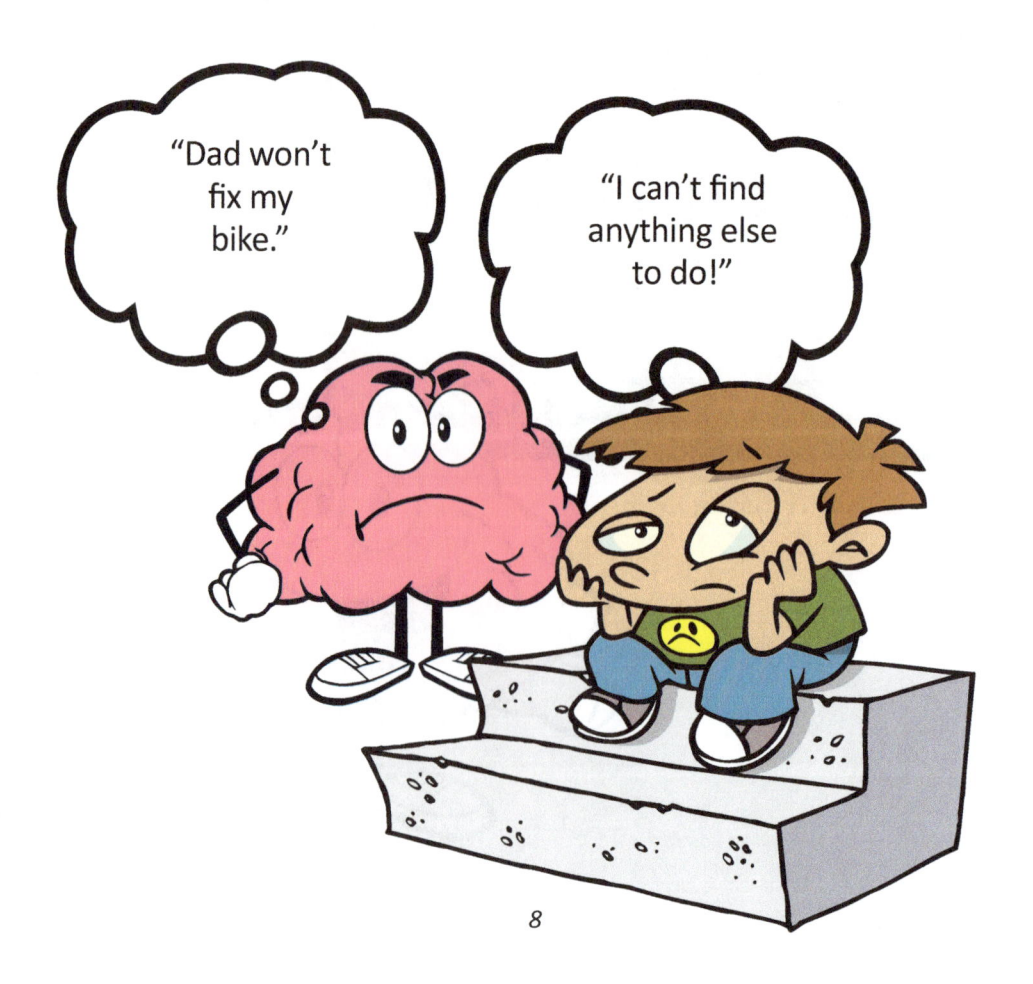

I need to find my brain-poline,

My brain trampoline.

I'll jump from black,

I'll jump from white,

And I'll jump to the rainbow in between.

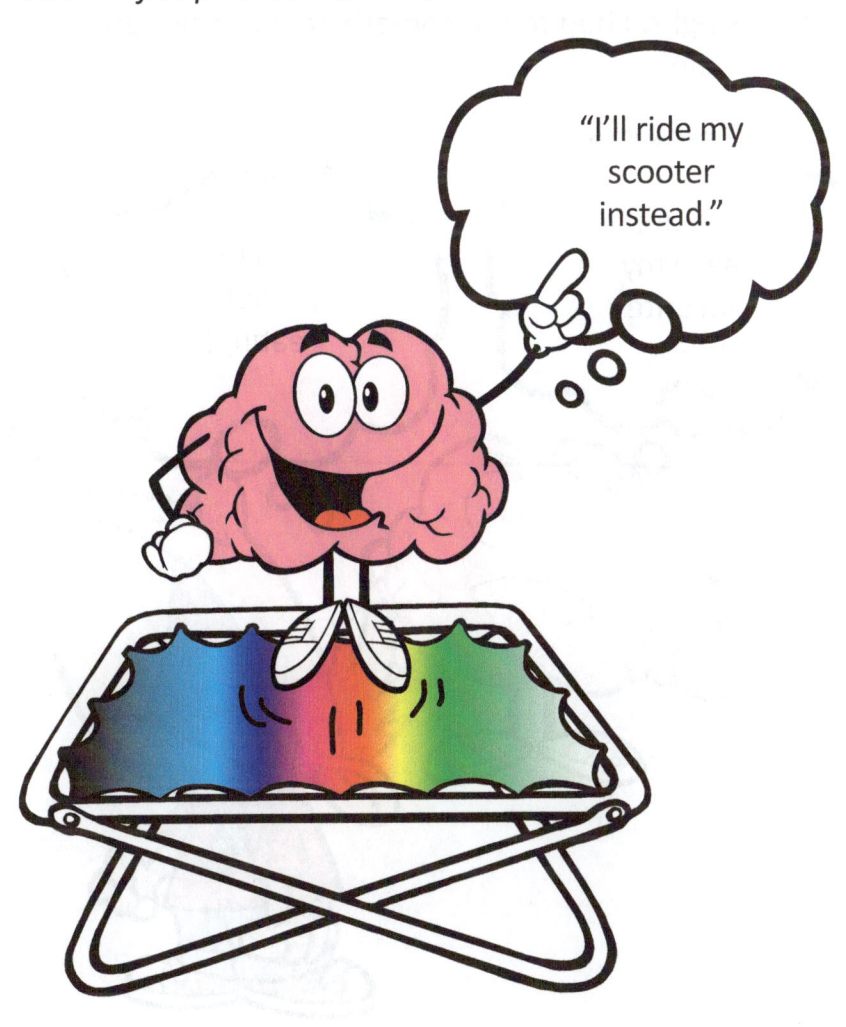

"I'll ride my scooter instead."

A Week of Switching, Shifting, and Stretching

On Monday, I wanted my favorite cheese for lunch. My favorite cheese, and that was it.

"If you don't have my favorite cheese, I'm not eating!"

Mom said, "You can't go all day without eating."

Uh oh!

Mom was right. I had to eat something. I was hungry. I needed help!

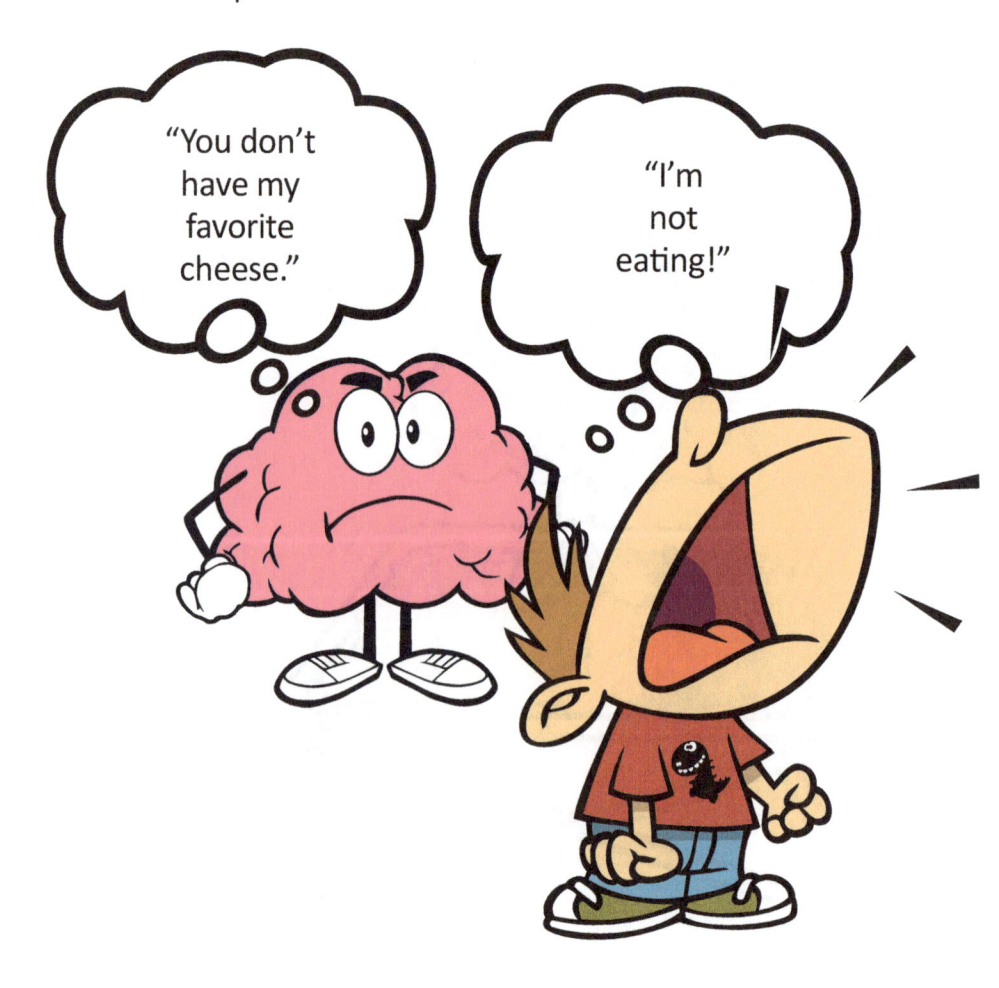

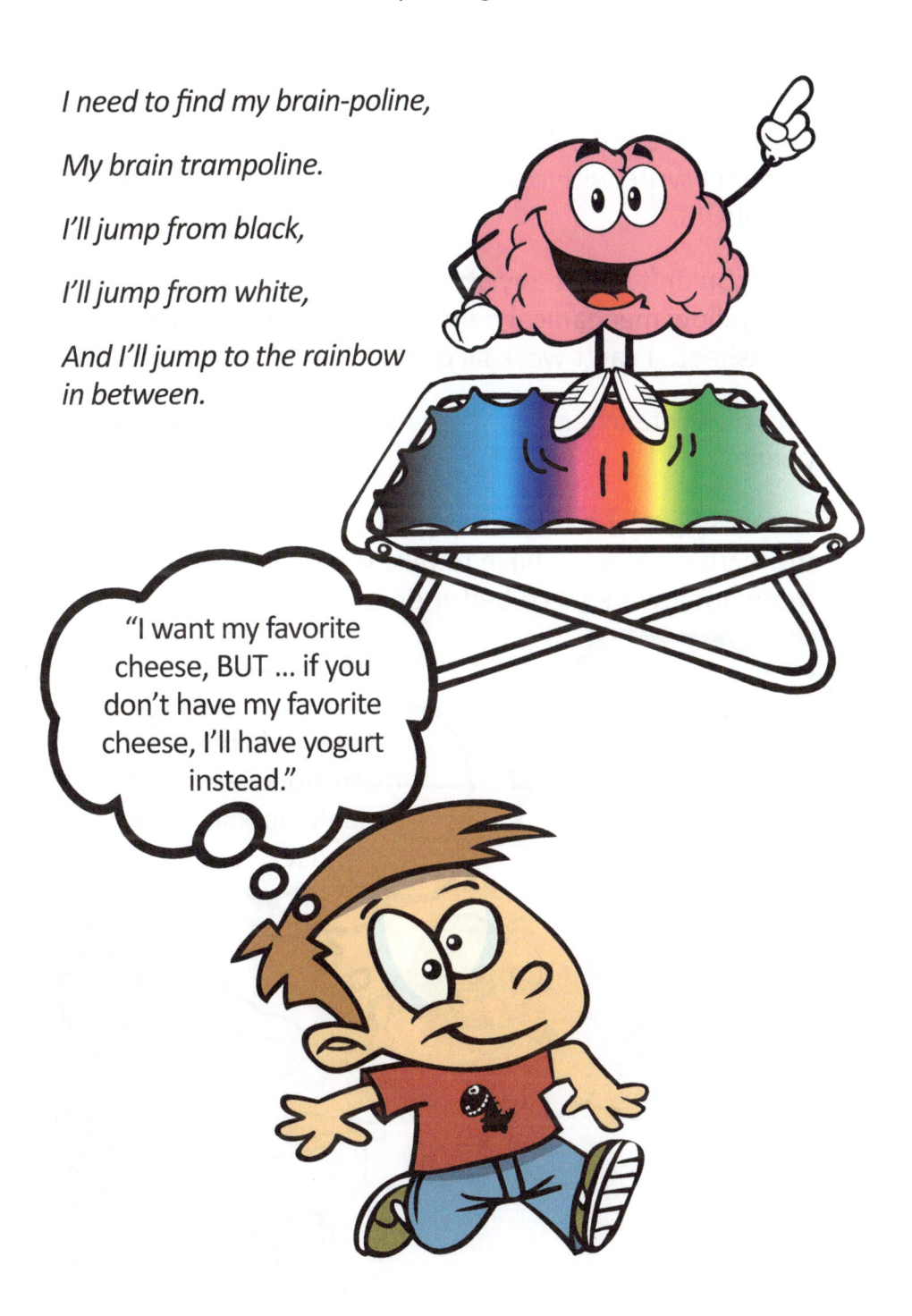

How to Make My Thinking More Flexible

I need to find my brain-poline,

My brain trampoline.

I'll jump from black,

I'll jump from white,

And I'll jump to the rainbow in between.

"I want my favorite cheese, BUT ... if you don't have my favorite cheese, I'll have yogurt instead."

A Week of Switching, Shifting, and Stretching

On Tuesday, I wanted to use my super-cool yellow mechanical pencil. I could not do my math worksheet if I didn't write with my super-cool yellow mechanical pencil.

But I couldn't find it anywhere. Oh, no! I lost my super-cool yellow mechanical pencil. I won't do my math worksheet. I can't work all day!

Uh oh! My teacher said, "You need to find your brain-poline."

She was right! I needed to stop and think. If I don't do my math in class, I'll have to take it home. I don't want more homework so I'd better do it now.

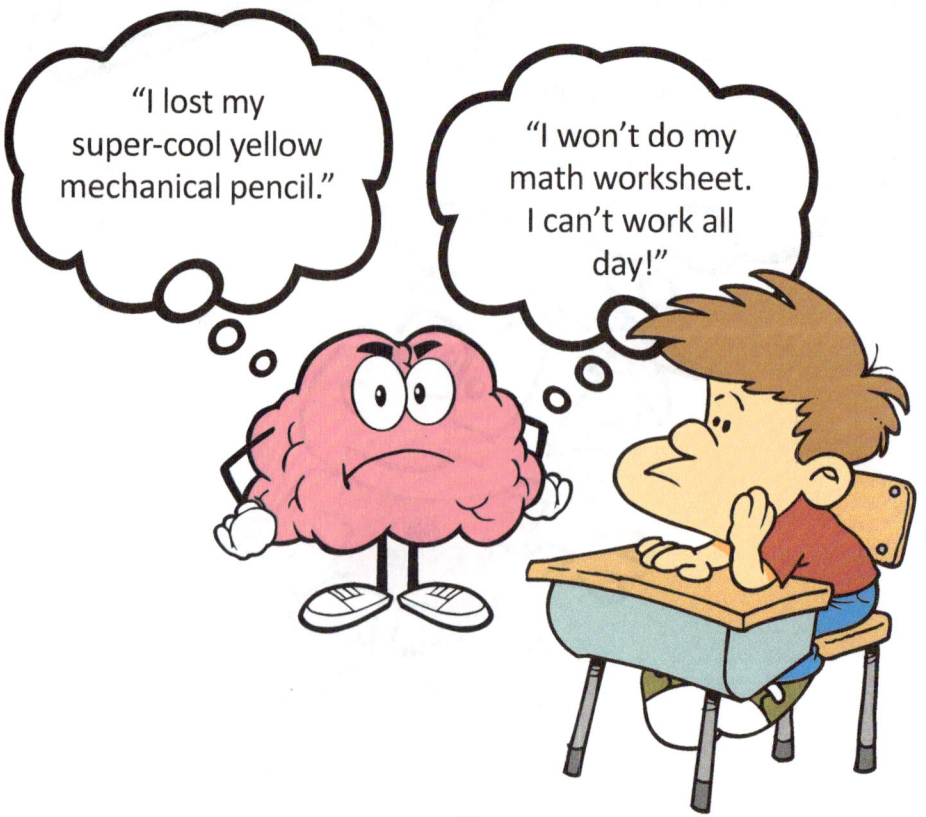

"I lost my super-cool yellow mechanical pencil."

"I won't do my math worksheet. I can't work all day!"

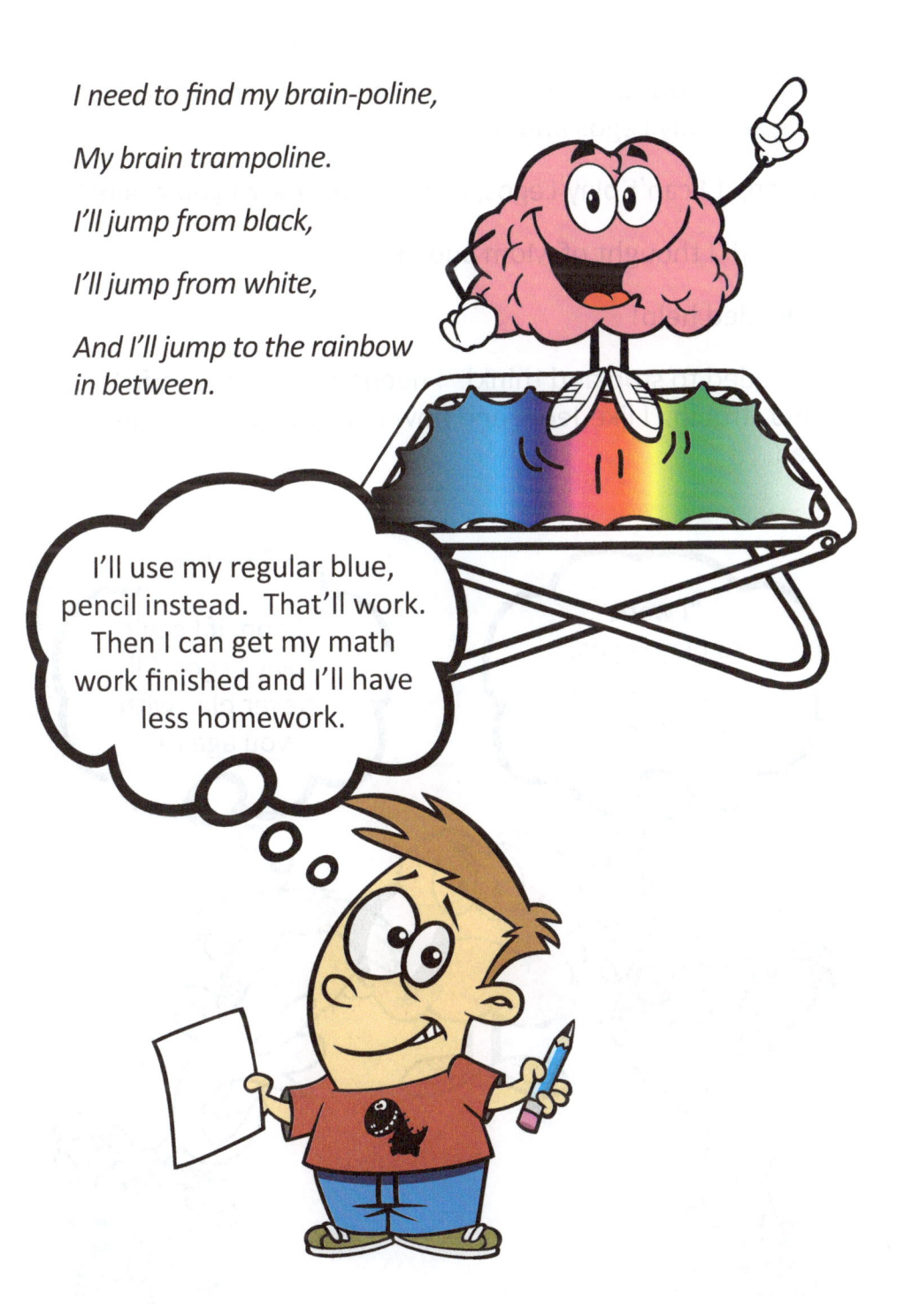

I need to find my brain-poline,

My brain trampoline.

I'll jump from black,

I'll jump from white,

And I'll jump to the rainbow in between.

I'll use my regular blue, pencil instead. That'll work. Then I can get my math work finished and I'll have less homework.

A Week of Switching, Shifting, and Stretching

On Wednesday, Jeon came over to play. I wanted to play Legos®, only Legos and nothing else!

"Jeon, if I can't play Legos, I'll never play with you again!"

Uh oh! I thought of Mom and I knew …

I needed help!

I needed to stop and think! I needed to switch, shift, and stretch. I like Jeon, and now I just made him super sad.

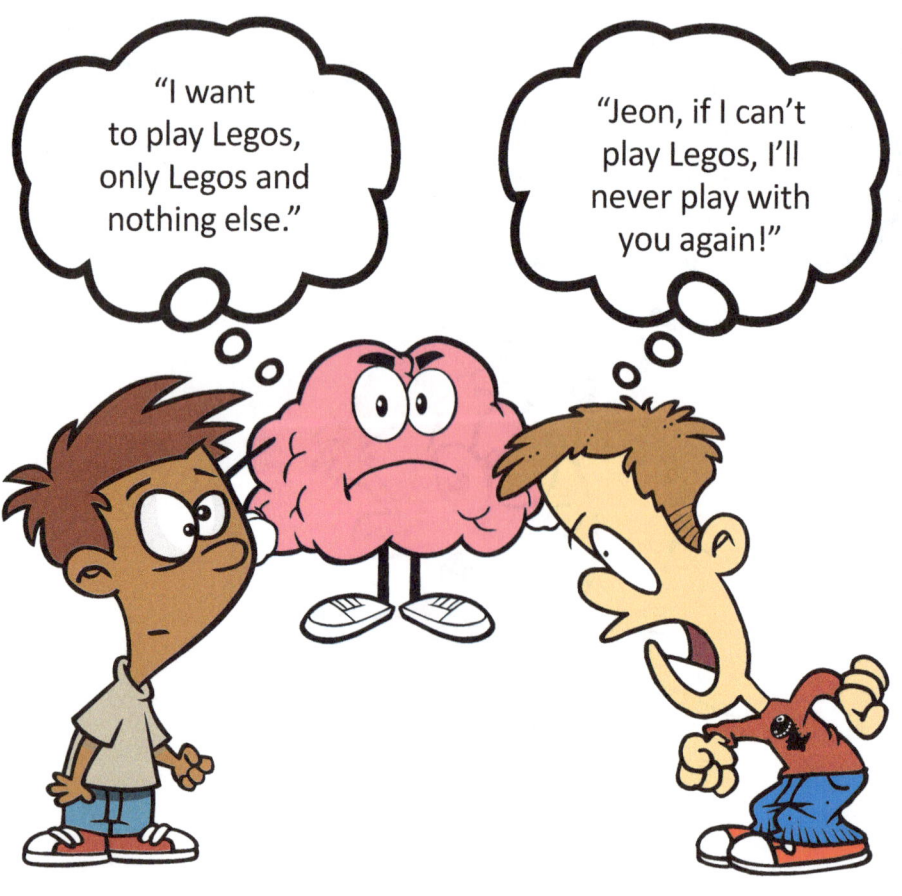

How to Make My Thinking More Flexible

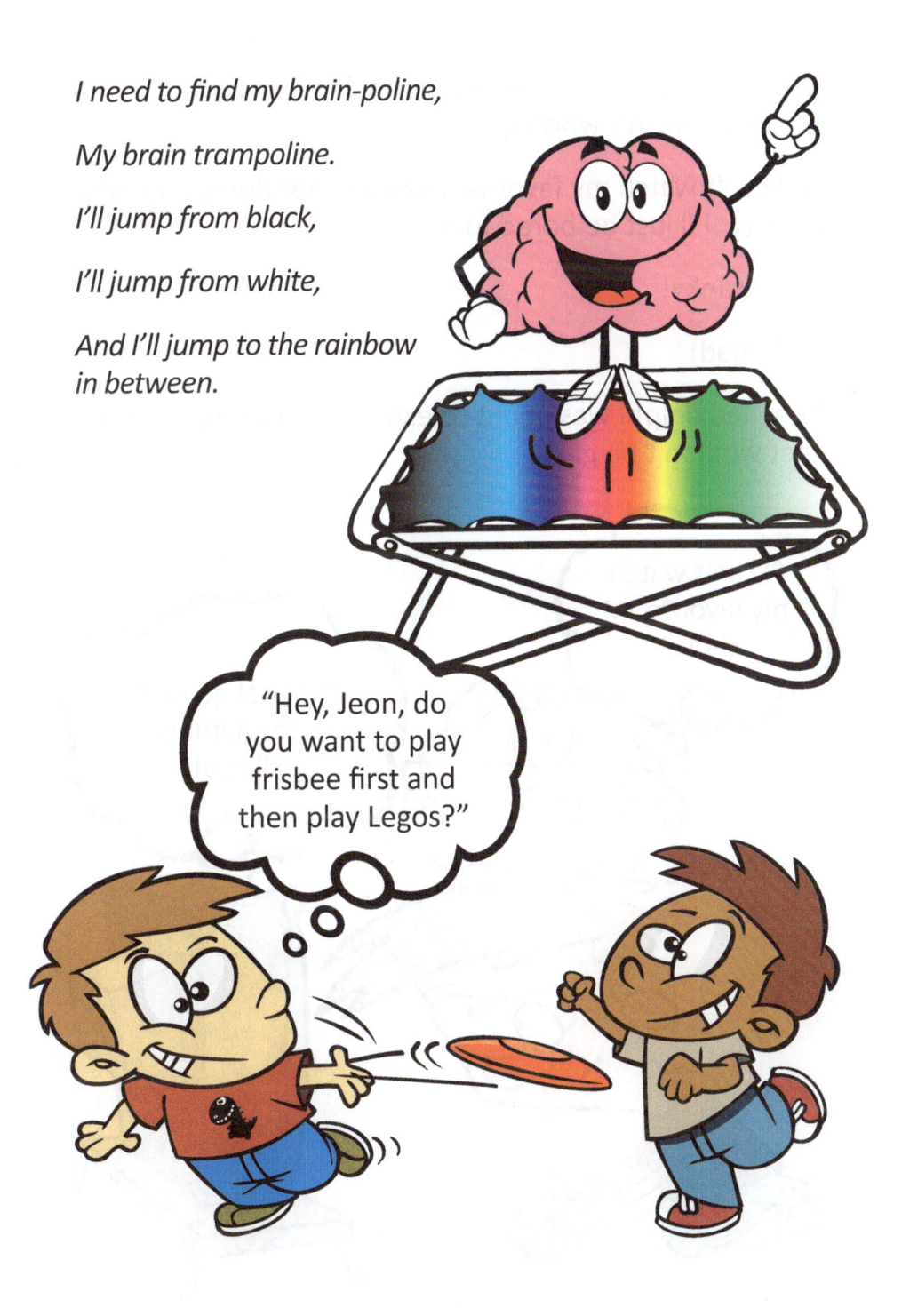

I need to find my brain-poline,

My brain trampoline.

I'll jump from black,

I'll jump from white,

And I'll jump to the rainbow in between.

"Hey, Jeon, do you want to play frisbee first and then play Legos?"

On Thursday, I wanted to watch my favorite show, but the cable wasn't working.

"If I can't watch my favorite show, I'm not doing anything all day. I'll just be bored forever."

I felt cranky!

I felt mad!

I needed help! I was about to explode like a volcano and that wouldn't be good.

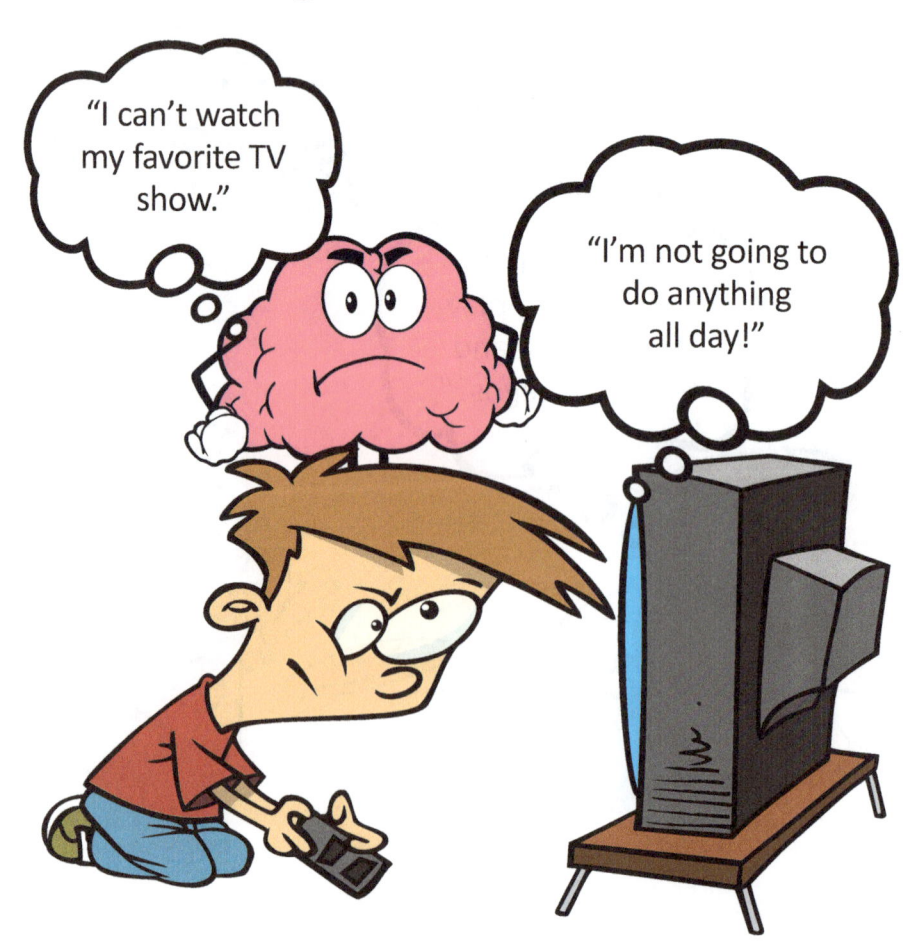

How to Make My Thinking More Flexible

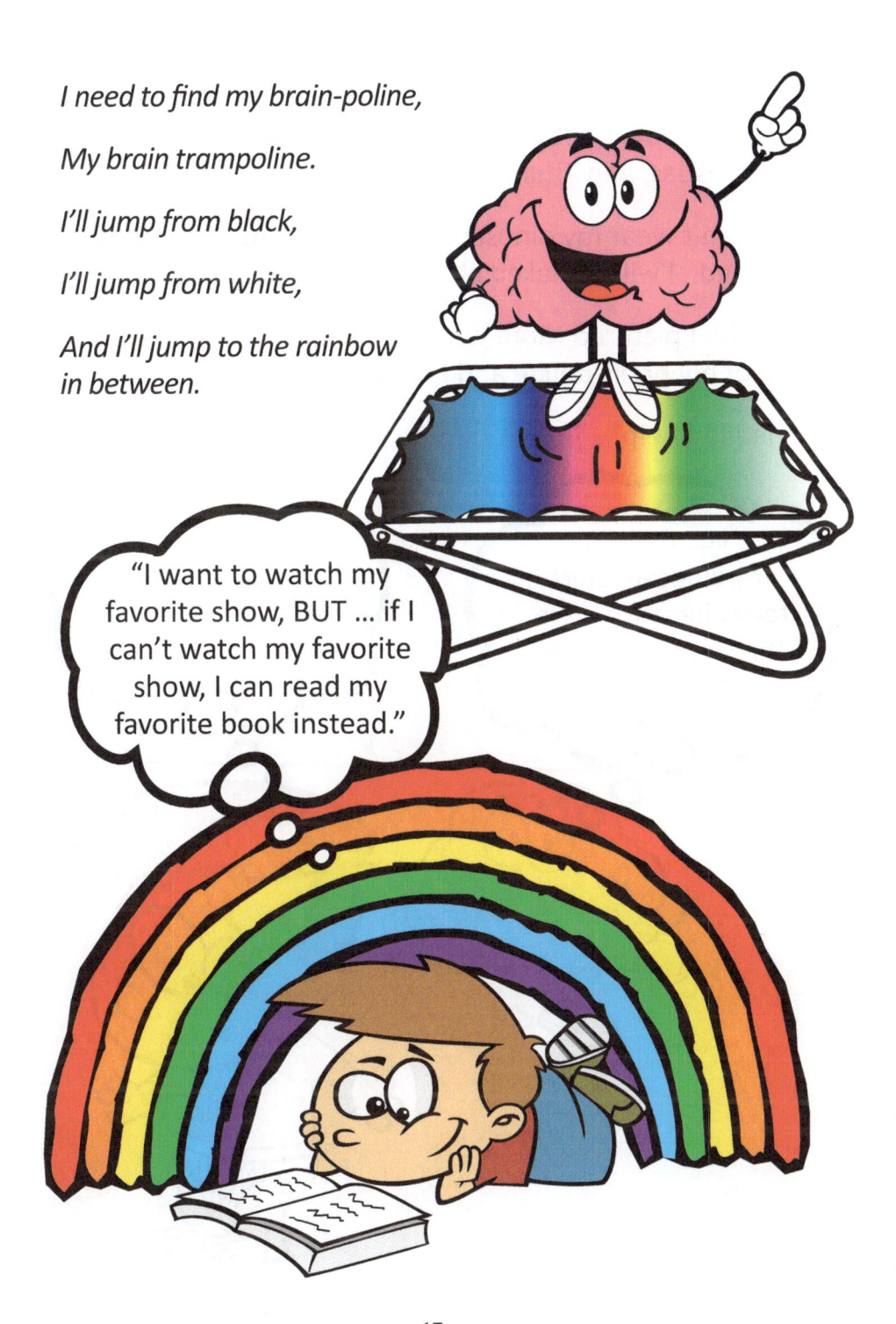

I need to find my brain-poline,

My brain trampoline.

I'll jump from black,

I'll jump from white,

And I'll jump to the rainbow in between.

"I want to watch my favorite show, BUT ... if I can't watch my favorite show, I can read my favorite book instead."

17

A Week of Switching, Shifting, and Stretching

On Friday, I wanted to wear my dinosaur shirt, but it was in the laundry because I had worn it Monday, Tuesday, Wednesday, and Thursday.

"If I can't wear my dinosaur shirt today, I'm not getting dressed. I will be naked all day."

Uh oh! I pictured Mom jumping up and down to remind me of my brain-poline and I knew:

I needed help!

"I can't wear my dinosaur shirt today because it's in the laundry. I'm not getting dressed."

"But then I'll be naked all day!"

How to Make My Thinking More Flexible

I need to find my brain-poline,

My brain trampoline.

I'll jump from black,

I'll jump from white,

And I'll jump to the rainbow in between.

"I really want my dinosaur shirt, BUT ... if I can't wear my dinosaur shirt, I'll wear my train shirt instead."

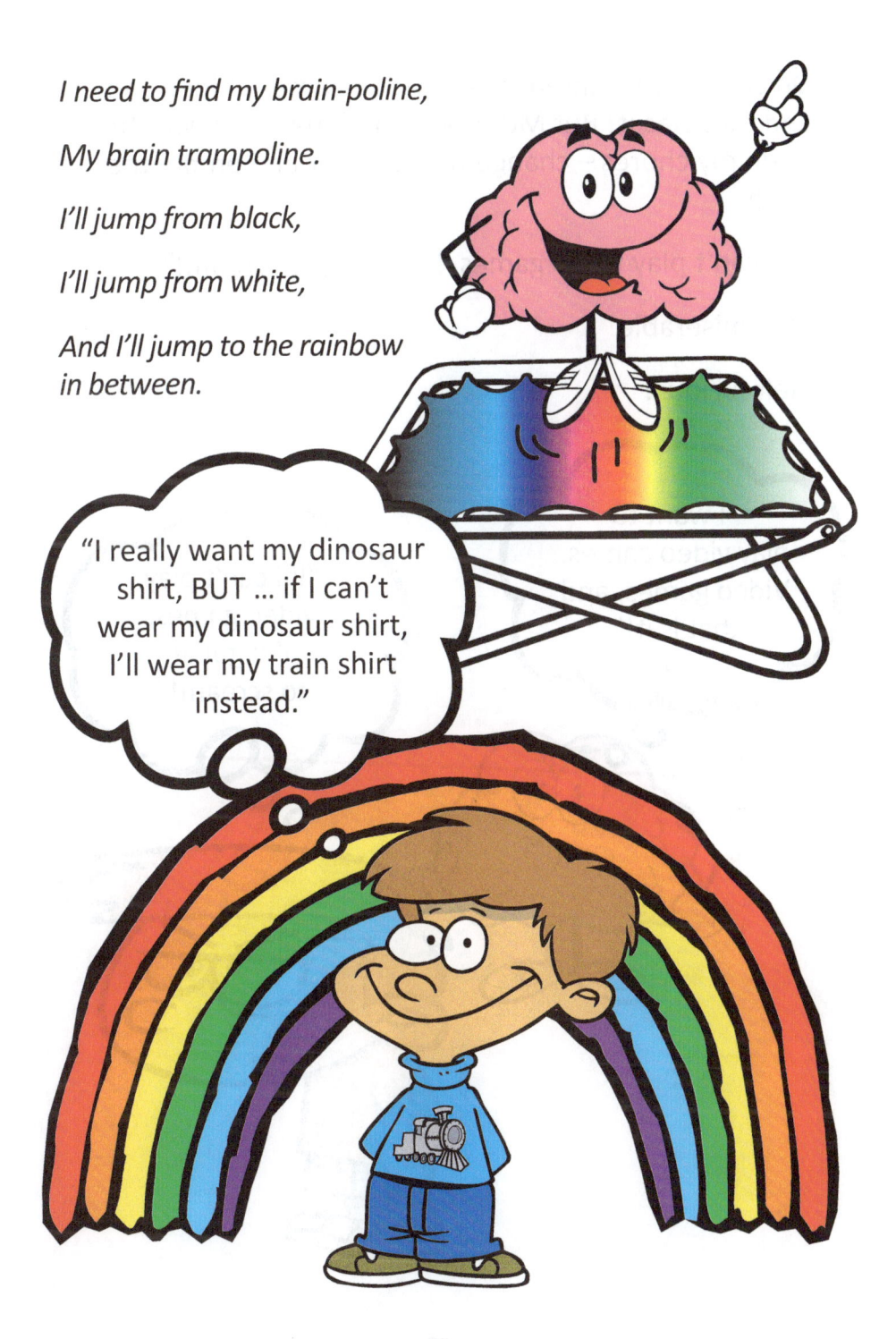

A Week of Switching, Shifting, and Stretching

On Saturday I wanted to play video games. Video games, and that was it! But Mom reminded me that it was time to do my chores – change the cat litter and empty the trash.

"If I can't play video games, I'm going to scream!"

I felt miserable!

I felt furious!

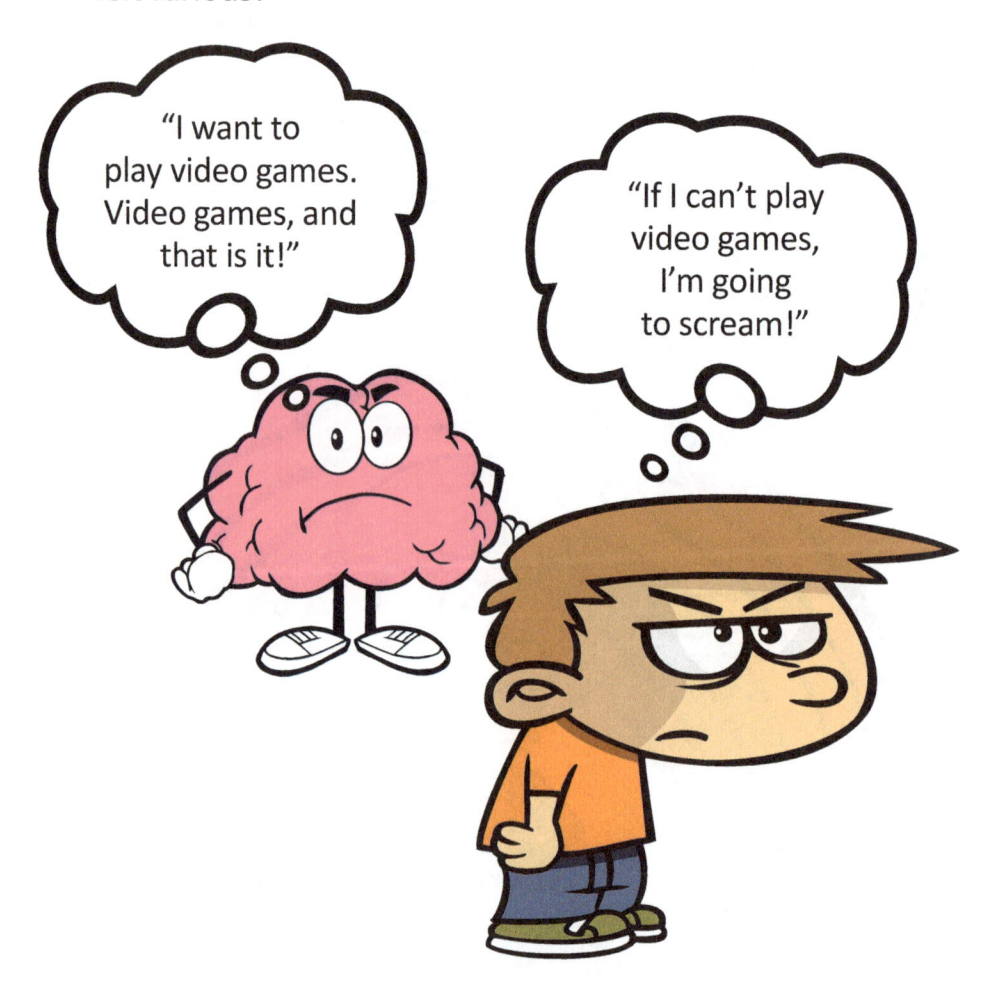

"I want to play video games. Video games, and that is it!"

"If I can't play video games, I'm going to scream!"

How to Make My Thinking More Flexible

Mom said,

"Go find your brain-poline,

Your brain trampoline.

You'll jump from black,

You'll jump from white,

And you'll jump to the wonderful rainbow in between."

"I really want video games, BUT ... I can do my chores first and then play video games."

FIRST... CHORES

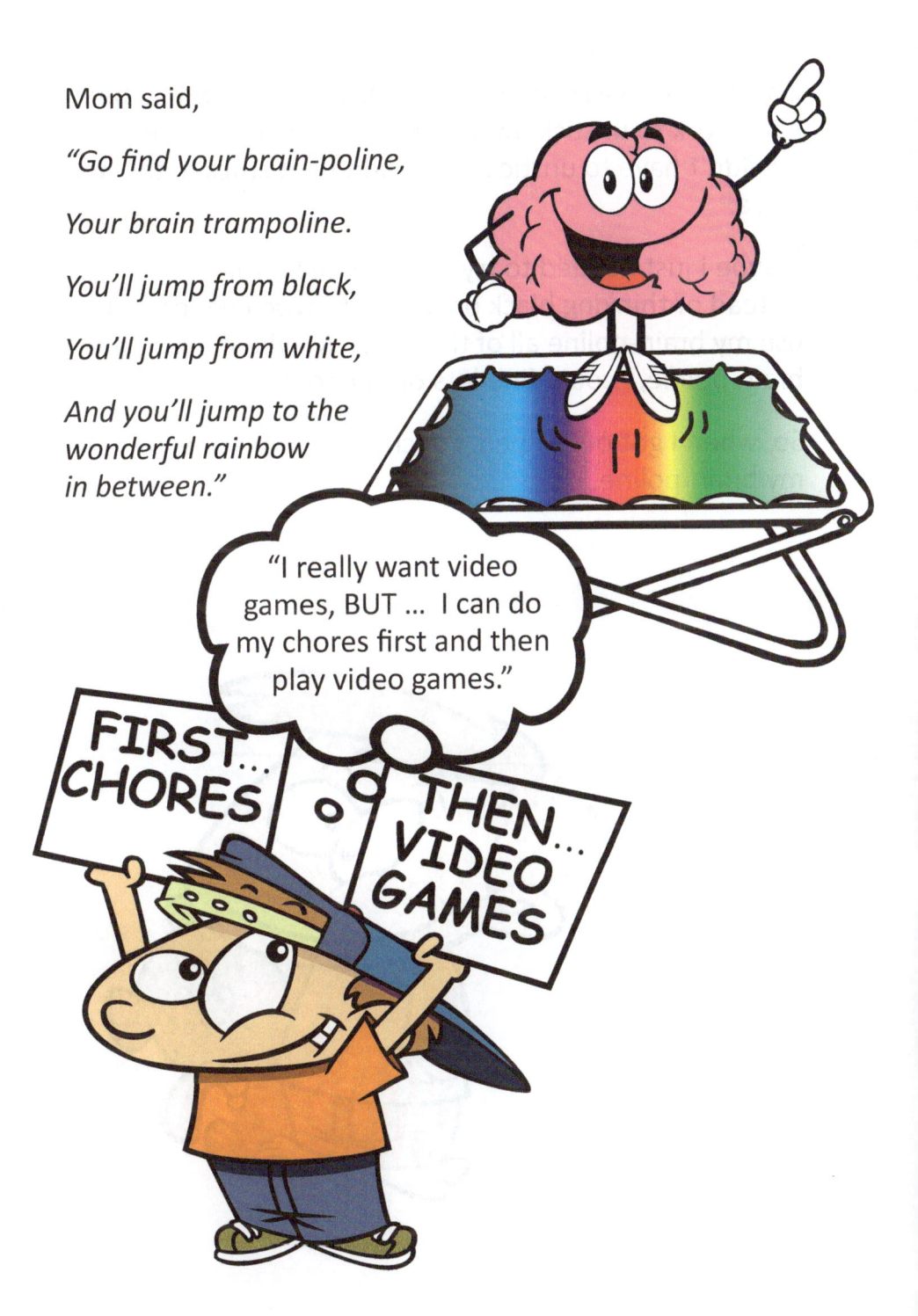

THEN... VIDEO GAMES

A Week of Switching, Shifting, and Stretching

On Sunday, I was exhausted, tired, worn out. It had been hard work to unstick my very stuck brain all week long. I wouldn't have to unstick it if it didn't get stuck in the first place.

Maybe I just needed to try more rainbow thinking instead of thinking black or white. Maybe I needed to use my brain-poline all of the time! Maybe if I used my brain-poline, I could find lots of rainbows.

So, when I got out of bed, I decided to jump directly on my brain-poline.

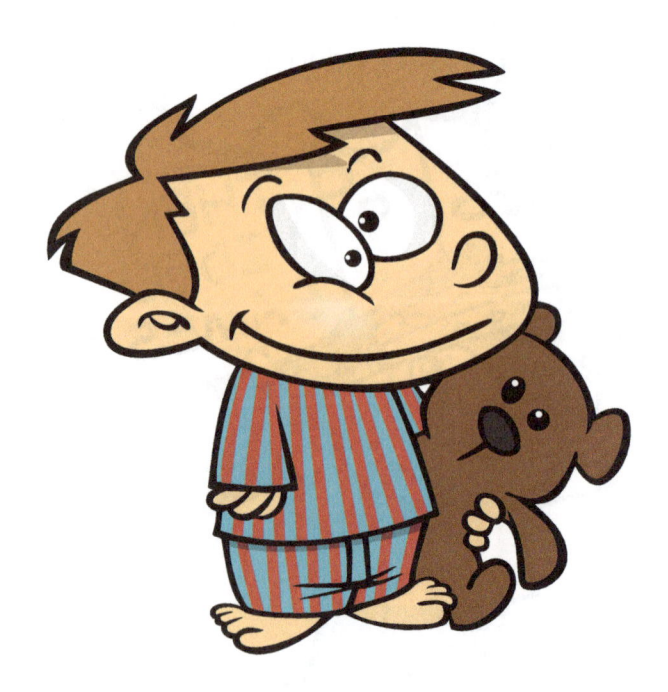

I jumped from black,

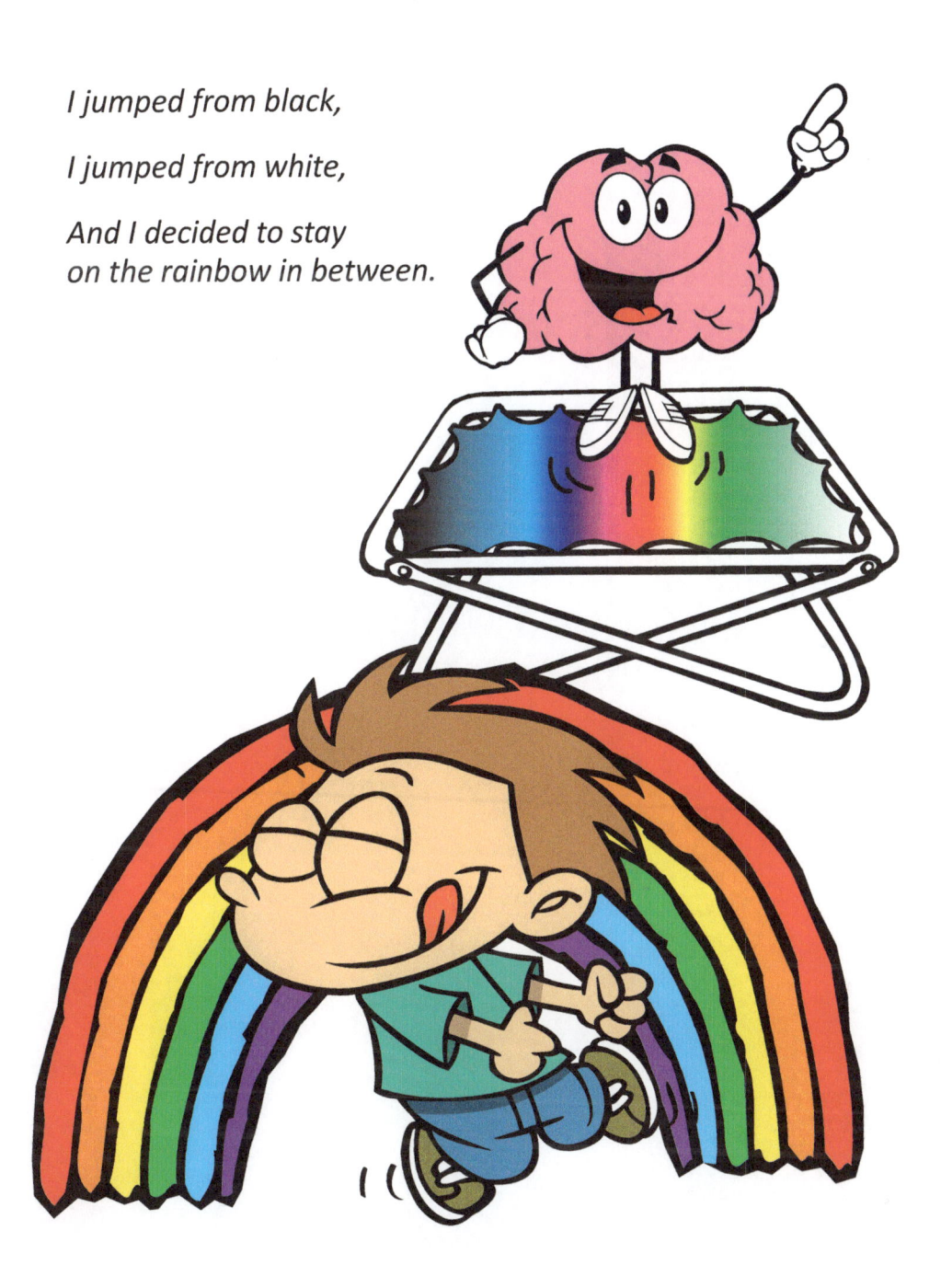

I jumped from white,

And I decided to stay
on the rainbow in between.

For Parents and Professionals

Jason's struggles are familiar to many of us. The ability to be flexible is a skill that can be challenging to learn and use. Jason becomes set in his ways because consistency and familiarity provide him with comfort. Using his super-cool yellow mechanical pencil, for example, potentially reduces his anxiety. However, the belief that he is unable to complete his work without it is a false assumption. It is a type of distorted thinking.

Throughout the story, the goal is for Jason to recognize that he has control over this distorted thinking. He must discover that he has the power to take control over his thoughts. Once he takes control of his thoughts, he has the power to be more flexible and, therefore, is able to interact more successfully with others.

Rigid thinking can limit a person greatly. Jason's rigid thinking could have damaged his relationship with his parents, sister, and friends, as well as his success in school. The ability to engage in flexible thinking is critical as it enables a child to experience the positive emotions that might come from a new pattern of thinking. The challenge is to help the child identify his current pattern of thinking and learn alternate ways to think about different situations.

The field of cognitive behavioral therapy (CBT) examines the relationship between thinking patterns, feelings, and behaviors.

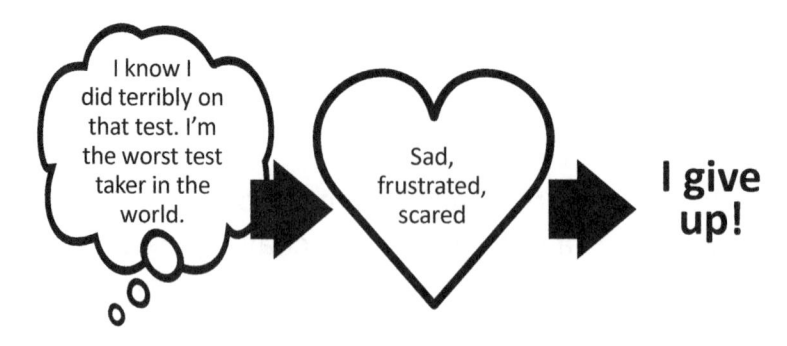

> I know I did terribly on that test. I'm the worst test taker in the world. ➡ Sad, frustrated, scared ➡ **I give up!**

The above example illustrates the link between our thoughts and feelings and subsequent actions. The thought (in the bubble) is an example of a thought distortion called "filtering" and "magnifying" (Briers, 2009). Filtering overlooks the good and positive in a situation and, therefore, has the same effect as magnifying, making negative thoughts and reactions seem bigger than they are. Both describe the black-and-white thinking in which Jason (and many others) engage.

CBT is one of the most empirically tested models of therapy, yielding positive results across ages and challenges.

Many of the programs and interventions described below are rooted in CBT and address the relationship between an individual's thoughts, emotions, and behaviors. Thoughts, emotions, and behaviors are inextricably linked. Positive thoughts lead to positive emotions and adaptive behaviors. Conversely, negative thoughts often lead to negative emotions and, ultimately, maladaptive behavior patterns.

For example, Jason believed that he was going to have a terrible day if he didn't wear his dinosaur shirt. This distorted thinking might lead to anxiety since his dinosaur shirt wasn't available. His anxiety might build to the point that he tantrums. This cycle of negative thoughts, behaviors, and emotions can be debilitating (Bearman & Weisz, 2012), restricting participation in activities and relationships.

In order to break this cycle, children have to be taught to examine their thinking, recognize distortions, and be flexible enough to change their patterns of thinking or, in the terminology used in this book, to become "rainbow thinkers."

Learning to Become a Flexible Thinker

Learning to be a rainbow thinker will increase positive thought patterns, positive emotions, and adaptive behaviors. Developing the ability to be a flexible thinker is critical since we live in a world that is often unpredictable on a good day, and downright disappointing on other days. For individuals who have trouble thinking in a flexible manner – switching, shifting, and stretching their thoughts – life can be pretty miserable. Often, people shy away from spending time with a person who is unable to think in a flexible way as such a person can be unpleasant to be around.

There are two major reasons why children (and adults) engage in black-and-white thinking, or cognitive distortions or thought distortions (Grohol, 2009). The first stems from *external experiences* we encounter in our lives. That is, environmental input shapes the way our brain processes information (Briers, 2009). For example, if we have had the unfortunate experience of being bitten by a dog, from the day it happened, whenever we see a dog, we may think, "danger." This thought process arises out of behavioral conditioning from one single bad experience (being bitten by a dog) without taking into account the fact that we have encountered lots of other dogs in the meantime that have been perfectly safe, loving creatures.

The second reason stems from *internal emotional experiences* that arise out of external experiences and impact the ways in which we view experiences (Briers, 2009). For example, if a child on the spectrum experiences continued failure in the social world, he may have negative feelings about social interactions and begin to think that he will always be unsuccessful in social situations. Such a belief system may lead to disengagement – why bother trying when you "know" that you will fail. "Nobody wants to be my friend" so I'm not going to the playground." In other words, this kind of thinking reinforces negative emotions and subsequent behavior (refusal to interact) and social interactions.

Black-and-white thinking is a rigid form of thinking that gives the illusion of control over situations over which children otherwise feel they have no control. Often, when people are anxious, their rigidity increases.

This rigidity becomes a kind of pseudo coping strategy as a way to remain in control. But in actuality, rigidity decreases control. Additionally, the irony in distorted thinking and rigidity is that they both increase anxiety rather than decreasing it.

Teaching children to be flexible thinkers is anything but easy. The following activities include evidence-based strategies and ideas that arose from the cognitive behavioral therapy literature. They are intended to facilitate, encourage, and "grow" flexible thinking in your child. Besides, they are simple, and sometimes even fun, require a minimum of materials and supplies, and can be used at home, at school, or in the community, with family or friends. I have used all of these activities as a clinician and have found that their experiential, visual nature increases children's engagement and learning.

What Will Happen If ...?

Brenda Smith Myles and Diane Adreon (2001) discuss the concept of "options" and "consequences" in a model called Situation-Options-Consequences-Choices-Strategies-Simulation (SOCCSS). SOCCSS, originally created by Jan Roosa, offers a model for practicing flexible thinking by encouraging individuals to examine cause and effect and ways in which to bring about a different, more positive outcome.

The following activity builds upon and incorporates SOCCSS as we work with children and adolescents to stop and think about the different options they have. If we can stop and think about different options, we can then practice flexible thinking to determine new options that might have more favorable outcomes.

What You Will Need

- Paper and pens or pencils (enough for everyone participating)

- Dry-erase board and markers (optional: one for each participant or just one for demonstration purposes for the person leading)

How to Play

In the first step of playing "What Will Happen If ...," tell the child that you are going to see if you can find your brain-poline and stretch your brain as far as it will go.

Emphasize that the game will be fun. You might even pose a challenge to the child to see who can make their brain stretch the farthest. (Please remember, children with autism spectrum and similar disorders become anxious in "win/lose" situations, so only make this into a competition if you are sure it will work with the child.) You can then be silly and pretend to stretch out your brain to get it ready.

Once you have introduced the game, describe a situation to the child. For example, you can say: "Imagine the following scenario: Allie, who is eight years old, went up to the lunch table in the cafeteria, and as soon as she sat down, all of the girls at the table began laughing. Allie immediately got up, threw her lunchbox down, and yelled, 'Why are you all laughing at me?'"

Why did Allie act the way she did? In other words, what assumptions did she make? What thoughts did she have in her head? You might draw a brain or thought bubbles and write in all of the different thoughts Allie might have had in her brain that made her act the way she did.

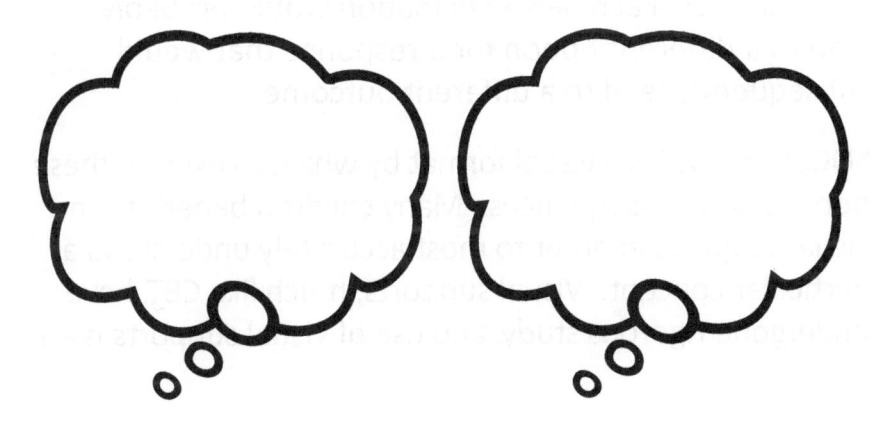

As adult facilitators, we recognize that Allie made an assumption about the girls' laughter and responded based on this assumption: *The girls were laughing at her.* It will be interesting to see if the child with whom you are interacting sees this the same way. Regardless, SOCCSS is a way in which to examine this assumption, discuss different ways to react, and work on flexible thinking in a similar situation.

It seems Allie made the assumption that the girls were laughing at her, which caused her to be sad and angry. Yelling, throwing her lunchbox, and walking away was the solution she chose to deal with the situation, based upon her assumptions and subsequent emotions. A caring adult could work with Allie to help her see that perhaps someone at the table had just told a joke that made everybody at the table laugh. Or perhaps the girls had made a bet that somebody might have chocolate in their lunchbox and somebody had just won the bet, causing them to break into laughter.

There are many other explanations for the girls breaking into laughter. Each new explanation would probably lead to a different option for a response that would subsequently lead to a different outcome.

SOCCSS provides a visual format by which to explore these options and consequences. Many children benefit from visual supports in order to most accurately understand a particular concept. Visual supports, much like CBT, have undergone rigorous study, and use of visual supports is an evidenced-based practice for working with children with autism spectrum disorders (Hume, 2008).

When using SOCCSS, you can either work on a scenario that has occurred in the past, that you anticipate will occur, or that you are actively dealing with. You might even work on a hypothetical situation such as the one with Allie. Sometimes it is easier for children to engage in activities if they involve a situation that did not actually happen to them. Thus, hypothetical situations have been found to be a useful way to work with children (van Nieuwenhuijzen, 2005). The objectivity involved can give children the emotional distance needed to practice flexible thinking.

The grid on the following page is an adaptation of SOCCSS and can be useful in helping children examine a situation, the feelings the situation triggered, and the possible ways in which to respond. The grid also provides the opportunity to examine the outcomes that might occur as a result of the ways in which a child responded.

A Week of Switching, Shifting, and Stretching

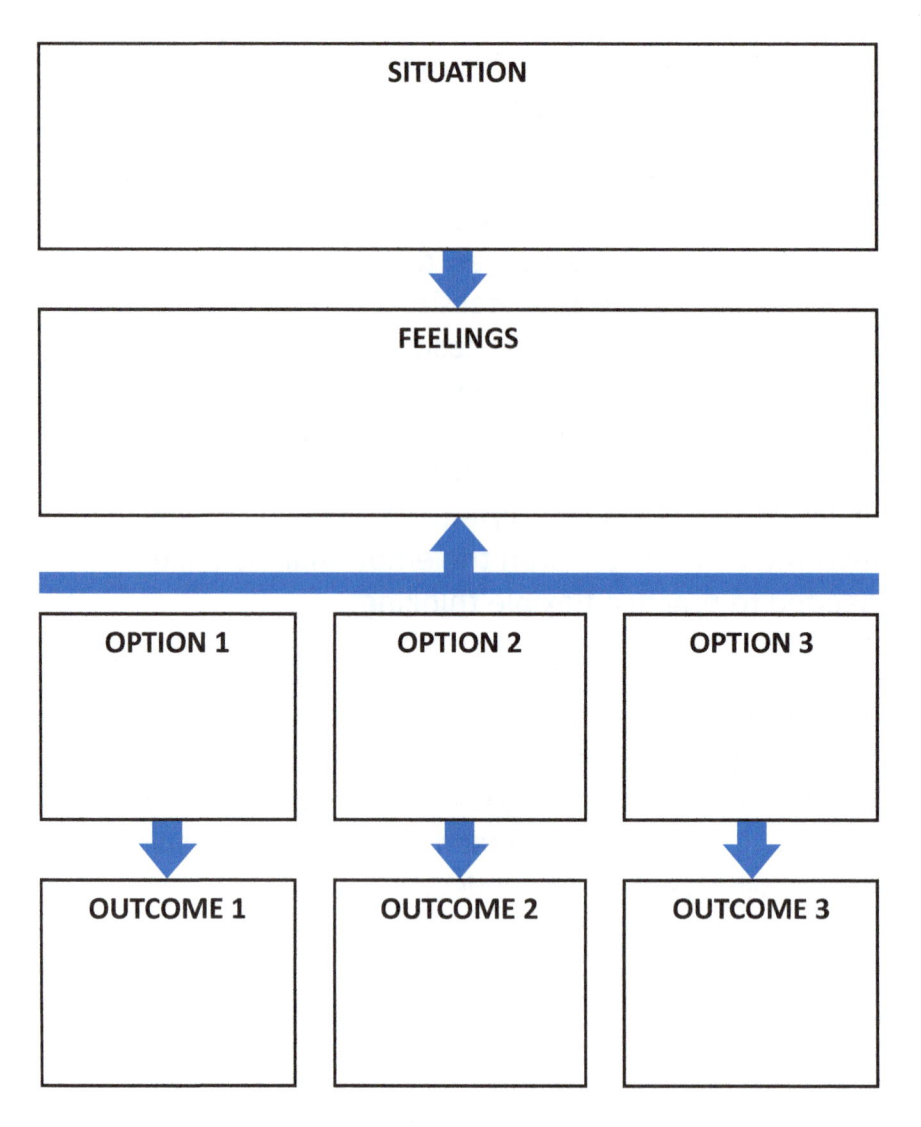

```
┌─────────────────────────────────────┐
│            SITUATION                │
│                                     │
│                                     │
└─────────────────────────────────────┘
                  ↓
┌─────────────────────────────────────┐
│            FEELINGS                 │
│                                     │
│                                     │
└─────────────────────────────────────┘
                  ↑
┌──────────┐  ┌──────────┐  ┌──────────┐
│ OPTION 1 │  │ OPTION 2 │  │ OPTION 3 │
│          │  │          │  │          │
│          │  │          │  │          │
└──────────┘  └──────────┘  └──────────┘
     ↓             ↓             ↓
┌──────────┐  ┌──────────┐  ┌──────────┐
│OUTCOME 1 │  │OUTCOME 2 │  │OUTCOME 3 │
│          │  │          │  │          │
│          │  │          │  │          │
└──────────┘  └──────────┘  └──────────┘
```

Whether you use this tool to address a current issue, a past situation, or a dilemma you anticipate may occur, it is critical to make sure the child is calm enough to "work" and engage in the process. If a child's behavior has escalated, he/she may not be able to problem solve and process the intervention (Collucci, 2011; Kerstein, 2008).

Additionally, Goleman (2008) focuses on the relationship between learning calming skills and the development of greater strength in the brain's circuits for managing stress. It would seem that this relationship is an important one on which to focus. If flexible thinking is stressful for a child, but he/she has learned ways to calm, might we assume that the ability to calm will ultimately lead to more frequent tolerance of flexible thinking demands?

As you work with your child to learn "rainbow thinking," it can also be helpful to assist him in generalizing this kind of flexible thinking by talking about other situations in which these particular options and outcomes might occur.

Can You Think of Three?

What You Will Need

- Some creative scenarios (see examples below)
- Paper and pens (enough for everyone participating)

How to Play

In the game *Can You Think of Three?*, the child can practice rainbow thinking in a non-intrusive and fun way. Present a situation and have the child think of three possible solutions. Here are some possible situations, but you can also make up your own scenarios.

You run out of dog food and you have to feed your dog.

You can:

1.

2.

3.

You are at a party, and the zipper on your pants breaks.

You can:

1.

2.

3.

You are hiking with your family, and you get lost.

You can:

1.

2.

3.

Working to think of multiple solutions to a particular "problem" encourages and practices flexible, or rainbow thinking.

How Many Games Can You Come up With?

What You Will Need

- A commercial game such as *Blink*® (Mattel), *Chutes and Ladders*® (Hasbro), a deck of cards, or *Othello*® (Mattel)

How to Play

The goals of this activity are to teach that (a) it is fun to use flexible thinking, (b) there are many different ways to play a game, (c) the experience of playing a game with another person is more fun than winning or losing, and (d) games can be fun even when others are in charge.

The first step is to introduce a particular game. You might say, "We're going to have a silly game day and see how many ways we can play this one game." Begin by playing the game the way it was designed to be played. After playing for a little while, take turns inventing new ways to play using the same materials from the game. For example, start out playing *Blink* traditionally and then play it as a matching game. You can then play it as a guessing game where someone holds the card up to their forehead (similar to the game *HedBanz*® [Spin Master Games]). When playing in this manner, one person holds a card up to her forehead and cannot look at what the card is saying. The other participants are supposed to provide clues so that the person can guess what card she has. The game may also be played as a simple pattern game in which you use the symbols on the cards to create different patterns across the table. The idea is to come up with as many different new games as possible based on the initial game.

Be Silly

What You Will Need

- Flexible thinking and good ideas regarding times of the day or activities in which you can practice being flexible, such as mealtimes, recess, driving, family games, bedtime, and seating in the classroom

How to Play

Create moments throughout the day or week when you have "silly" times. Let the child know that these are times when you are going to be "silly" and try something different.

1. Switch seats at the dinner table for a night.
2. Switch the desk at which you will sit that day (with the teacher's permission).
3. Drive home a different way from school.
4. Model flexibility by drinking out of a different cup than you typically do, brushing your teeth in the kitchen instead of the bathroom, having lunch food for breakfast, or having breakfast for lunch.
5. Sit in a different place on the couch than you usually do.
6. Walk a different route to a specials class.
7. Eat dinner in the dining room instead of the kitchen.
8. Encourage the child to jump on one leg down the hall instead of walking.

9. Play on a different piece of equipment on the playground.
10. Use a pen instead of a pencil.
11. Carry your backpack on your left shoulder instead of your right shoulder or your right shoulder instead of your left shoulder.
12. Sit at a different table in the cafeteria.
13. Read a book that you never considered reading before.
14. Talk to a teacher or peer at school about something you know they are interested in and not what you like most.

In short, change things around, be silly, model flexibility, and talk about flexibility. To model flexibility, you can narrate moments when you are attempting rainbow thinking. You can talk about how you were planning to make bean chili for dinner but forgot to buy the beans. You might say something like, "Oh well. I forgot the beans. No big deal. We'll have macaroni and cheese instead. I'm using flexible thinking, or rainbow thinking."

Using Your Brain-Poline

What You Will Need

- A picture of a brain-poline (see page 9 of this book)
- Your singing voice

How to Play

Anticipate times when the child may have trouble thinking flexibly and remind her to use her brain-poline. Talk about times when she had trouble being flexible in the past and ways she could have used her brain-poline. Together, "catch" others who are having trouble being flexible and talk about how they need to use their brain-poline. You might keep a copy of the brain-poline in your pocket so that you can pull it out to show the child. You can also keep a picture on the refrigerator to remind the whole family to use their brain-poline or keep a picture of a brain-poline on the board at school. It can also be helpful to have the child draw a picture of what her brain-poline looks like. As you "catch" each other being flexible, or conversely, having trouble using your brain-poline, you can sing the following song (actually, it is more of a chant) together as a reminder and a reinforcer.

The Brain-Poline Song

I need to find my brain-poline,

My brain trampoline.

I'll jump from black,

I'll jump from white,

And I'll jump to the rainbow in between.

Recognition and Praise

What You Will Need

- A copy of this book

How to Play

Praise the child every time you see or hear about moments when he used flexible or rainbow thinking. Point out how well he used his brain-poline; that is, the times when he was able to switch, stretch, or shift his thinking and use rainbow thinking. It is important to be specific with praise; otherwise, it loses its meaning and impact. For example, say, "I like how you used your brain-poline when you couldn't find your favorite red shirt and wore a blue shirt instead. Nice rainbow thinking!" instead of, "I like how you used your brain-poline."

You might even use a reinforcement system for a brief period of time. You can draw your own brain-poline and encourage your child to put a sticker, smiley face, check mark, or tally mark on it each time he/she uses his/her brain-poline. This will reinforce flexible thinking. The more specific you are with praise, the more your child will begin to understand the concept of flexible thinking.

A Week of Switching, Shifting, and Stretching

5-Point Scale: Feelings and Their Triggers

What You Will Need

- A 5-point scale (see below)

Rating	How I Feel	Cause	Reaction
5			
4			
3			
2			
1			

Activity

The Incredible 5-Point Scale by Kari Dunn Buron and Mitzi Curtis (2012) has been found to be a very effective tool for teaching children social and emotional concepts in a concrete, visual manner. In particular, it can be very helpful for assisting a child in examining triggers, emotion intensity, and developing better coping strategies.

The following are examples of situations where use of *The Incredible 5-Point Scale* can be effective:

1. Max is a six-year-old student who just began first grade. He tends to refuse to participate in activities in new environments. Rather than acting out, he typically shuts down and becomes unresponsive. A 5-point scale can help Max understand the intensity of his emotion, the negative thoughts he is experiencing, and ways to cope and respond that are more successful than his typical way of shutting down.

Max's Scared Scale

Rating	How I Feel	Cause	Reaction
5	Terrified	If my teacher becomes upset with me because I won't try it.	I hide in the bathroom in the hallway and refuse to come out.
4	Horrified	If my teacher tries to get me to do something new.	I leave the room.
3	Very scared	If I am asked to try something new.	I won't talk at all.
2	Scared	If I think I will have to try something new.	I am more quiet.
1	A little bit scared	On days that are not ordinary.	I still play with my friends but watch for new things.

2. Janie is an eight-year-old girl who is homeschooled. Whenever her mother changes the schedule for the day, Janie becomes angry and yells at her. She often ends up in a full-blown rage. Using the 5-point scale will help Janie understand the trigger that causes her behavior, the intensity of her emotion, and ways in which to handle this trigger in the future.

Janie's Anger Scale

Rating	How I Feel	Cause	Reaction
5	Furious	If Mom completely changes the schedule for the day.	I might yell and rage.
4	Angry	If we have to go to a doctor's in the middle of a lesson.	Whine, raise my voice.
3	Somewhat angry	If Mom asks me to try harder on something new.	Whine, get somewhat angry.
2	A little angry	If I don't understand something.	Ask for help.
1	Okay	On a day that is mostly typical.	I still play with my friends but watch for new things.

Trigger Me!

What You Will Need

- Paper and markers (enough for everyone participating)
- Pictures that show the relationship between cause and effect, such as the ones below

How to Play

Spend time teaching the child what the word *trigger* means. Triggers can include events that cause an emotional reaction (happiness, excitement) such as winning a game, or a sensory reaction (feeling sick to the stomach, headache) from the smell of burnt toast. It is important to help the child investigate the things that act as triggers and cause problems. This includes exploring triggers in all the environments in which the child spends time (school, home, the mall, a relative's house, etc.).

The following are suggestions for ways to teach the child the relationship between cause and effect. If cause and effect is not understood, children may not realize the negative impact their rigid thinking has on others. Additionally, children may not realize the positive impact their flexible thinking has on others. Finally, they may not realize the events, experiences, and sensations in their lives that cause them to feel a particular way.

How to Make My Thinking More Flexible

Stimuli and Triggers Can Cause Feelings – What Does This Really Mean?

Many of the worksheets in the rest of this book ask you to think about feelings a person may experience as a result of stimuli he has encountered.

Facilitators: You may be thinking, "How am I going to explain *stimuli* to the child?"

Explorers: You may be thinking, "What does *stimuli* really mean?"

Let's take a look at what the word *stimuli* means. First of all, *stimuli* is the plural *stimulus*; that is, it indicates that we are dealing with more than one. If you look up the word *stimulus* in Roget's New Millennium Thesaurus (http://thesaurus.reference.com/help/faq/roget.html), you may find such words as *bang, catalyst, kick, incitement, wave maker, impulse, spark plug*.

I find it helpful to think of a stimulus as a "wave maker." If you throw a large rock into the water, it creates a wave. The rock is the **stimulus** that **caused** the wave.

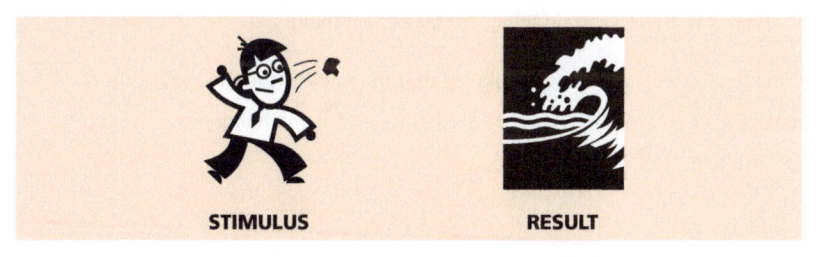

STIMULUS   **RESULT**

Similarly, a strong smell of perfume may cause you to feel sick:

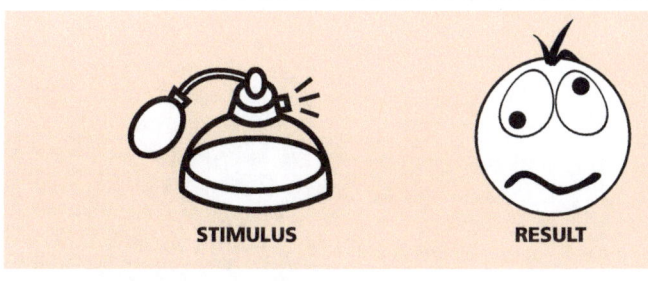

STIMULUS   **RESULT**

Note. Pages 47-51 are from L. H. Kerstein, *My Sensory Book: Working Together to Explore Sensory Issues and the Big Feelings They Can Cause*, 2008, Shawnee Mission, KS: AAPC Publishing. Used with permission.

But the smell of newly baked chocolate chip cookies may make you feel happy (and hungry):

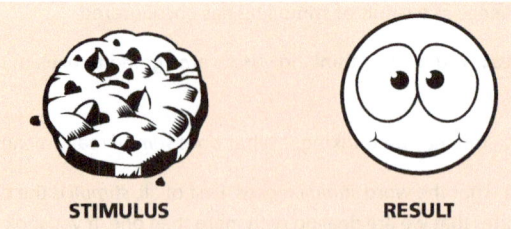

STIMULUS   **RESULT**

So, a stimulus is something that CAUSES you to feel a certain way, think a certain thing, or do a certain thing. And, *stimuli are more than one stimulus.* So . . . you may smell the chocolate chip cookies, feel happy and hungry, think, "that smells delicious," and run right into the kitchen to get one to eat. Yum!

Stimuli are also called TRIGGERS. A TRIGGER is also something that causes you to feel a certain way, think a certain thing, or do a certain thing.

Using the example above, we could say that the smell of the chocolate chip cookies *TRIGGERED* you to *FEEL* happy and hungry so you *ATE* one.

How to Make My Thinking More Flexible

Facilitators: Many of the worksheets throughout this book will ask you to help the child explore a variety of stimuli or triggers and the feelings they might cause. It may be useful to explore the different feelings by acting them out, thinking of situations that have caused feelings, or reading some books listed and discussing the different feelings feelings encountered in the books. Take a moment to help the child identify triggers in her everyday life and the feelings they cause her. The triggers can be sensory related or be related to other daily events. You can do this using the Trigger Chart.

Explorers: As you can see, you will be asked to talk about feelings on some of the worksheets in the book since *STIMULI* and *TRIGGERS* can cause lots of different feelings. I know this may not be your favorite topic of conversation, but it is really helpful to figure out your feelings so you can decide what to do with them. Understanding your feelings and controlling them is not easy, but it is far better to **take control** of your feelings than to let your feelings control you.

If you are having trouble figuring out this mysterious world of feelings, you may want to ask an adult such as a parent, teacher, or member of your family to help you. You may think, "Those are way too young for me" and you may be right. But they can help you make a little more sense of feelings. I bet your parents still have your old children's books somewhere in the house, or perhaps they can help you check some out of the library.

Once you feel you understand the world of feelings, you can describe (and draw) feelings on the next page and write things that may cause people to have those feelings. Take a moment and write down triggers in your everyday life and identify the feelings they cause you to feel. The triggers can be sensory related or simply things that happen in your life. You can write this on the Trigger Chart.

A Week of Switching, Shifting, and Stretching

A Quick Look at the Things That Trigger My Feelings

I think _____ means _____
         feeling   describe the feeling

_____. It seems people usually feel this way

when the following happens: _____
                              name things that can trigger this feeling

_____.

Draw a picture of feeling

I think _____ means _____
         feeling   describe the feeling

_____. It seems people usually feel this way

when the following happens: _____
                              name things that can trigger this feeling

_____.

Draw a picture of feeling

I think _____ means _____
         feeling   describe the feeling

_____. It seems people usually feel this way

when the following happens: _____
                              name things that can trigger this feeling

_____.

Draw a picture of feeling

How to Make My Thinking More Flexible

Trigger Chart

Trigger	Feelings (positive or negative)	Stress Rating (1-5)
My sister knocked over my blocks.	Angry, Furious, Upset	5

Facilitators and Explorers: This chapter provided an introduction to the idea that we all have many different feelings (positive and negative) that can impact us each day. We also looked at the fact that there are stimuli or triggers that can cause us to feel, think, or do certain things. Finally, we began to explore the INTENSITY of feelings.

Using Your Five Senses to Understand Your World and Your Feelings

What You Will Need:

- Copies of page 54 (enough for everyone participating)
- Paper and pencil or pen for all participants

How to Play

We are all faced with having to filter the myriad pieces of information that come at us at all times. This information can be environmental, such as the sound of the siren of a fire truck or the smell of Asian food from a nearby restaurant, or internal, such as a stomachache or a cold. Some of us smoothly focus on the relevant information in our environment, such as a teacher talking or the words we are reading in a book, while filtering out the irrelevant information that also comes our way. Others have challenges in this area and find themselves distracted by irrelevant information, such as the hum of lights or a headache and, therefore, unable to focus on the relevant information.

It is very anxiety-provoking to have trouble focusing on the things that are most important, such as a test review versus the cars driving by the classroom window. In an attempt to cope, children may experience a lot of negative or distorted thinking. For example, a child who has trouble filtering out irrelevant noise in the classroom may begin to think, "I'm never going to do well on that test. I can't concentrate."

One activity that can help children to develop a better understanding of their sensory systems involves taking a "sensory tour" of their environment and thereby encourage them to pay attention to and understand what they see, hear, smell, taste, and touch in their environments. In the following, we take such a tour as it relates to hearing. You can then talk about the impact of these forms of sensory input on their moods, on their thinking, and on the ways their bodies regulate (Wilbarger & Wilbarger, 1991); that is, the level of alertness they experience. For example, Eeyore moves very slowly/probably too slowly, Tigger moves very fast/probably too fast, and Pooh moves "just right." Sensory input can impact the speed at which our bodies and brains are functioning.

When our level of alertness is "just right," our ability to focus, concentrate, participate, and comprehend increases. There are many ways to strive to reach optimal levels. These include chewing gum, drinking a beverage, chewing on pens or pencils, eating, or pacing. Most people, at some point in their day, need to utilize some kind of strategy in order to reach their "just right" level of arousal. We, as adults, typically know what helps us. Children don't. It is our job to help children find the strategies that ultimately help them reach their optimal level of functioning.

A Week of Switching, Shifting, and Stretching

What I Can Hear with My Ears

Stimuli	Feelings		Strategies
	Positive Feelings	Negative Feelings	

When I hear something that bothers me, my body goes: (circle one)

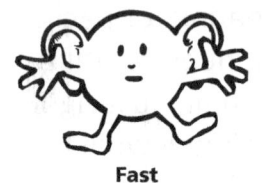

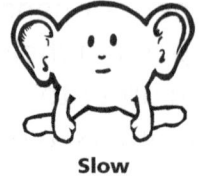

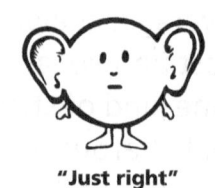

Fast   Slow   "Just right"

From L. H. Kerstein, *My Sensory Book: Working Together to Explore Sensory Issues and the Big Feelings They Can Cause*, 2008, Shawnee Mission, KS: AAPC Publishing. Used with permission.

Summary

The use of concrete tools can help increase the ability to be flexible thinkers and engage in rainbow thinking rather than black-and-white thinking. Flexible thinking is critical for being able to manage everyday changes and challenges. Many adults tend to shy away from challenging our children's black-and-white thinking for fear of meltdowns and tantrums. While understandable, shying away from teaching this important skill often leads children down paths of negative thinking and negative feelings. Although the process may be painful at first, tackling challenges with black-and-white thinking and finding your child's brain-poline is one of the most important skill you can teach your child – for a lifetime.

May we all find our brain-polines and stay flexible rather than rigid and stuck and, therefore, find life more fun and interesting!

References

Bearman, S. K., & Weisz, J. R. (2012). Cognitive behavioral therapy for children and adolescents: An introduction. In E. Szigethy, J. R. Weisz, & R. I. Findling (Eds.), *CBT for children and adolescents* (pp. 1-28). Washington, DC: American Psychiatric Publishing.

Briers, S. (2009). *Brilliant cognitive behavioral therapy.* London, UK: Pearson Education Limited.

Buron K. D., & Curtis, M. (2012). *The incredible 5-point scale: Assisting students with autism spectrum disorders in understanding social interactions and controlling their emotional responses* (2nd ed.). Shawnee Mission, KS: AAPC Publishing.

Collucci, A. (2011). *Big picture thinking: Using central coherence theory to support social skills.* Shawnee Mission, KS: AAPC Publishing.

Goleman, D. (2008). Introduction. In L. Lantieri (Ed.), *Building emotional intelligence: Techniques for cultivating inner strength in children* (pp. 1-4). Boulder, CO: Sounds True.

Grohol, J. (2009). *15 common cognitive distortions.* Retrieved from http://psychcentral.com/lib/2009/15-common-cognitive-distortions/

Hume, K. (2008). *Overview of visual supports*. Chapel Hill, NC: The University of North Carolina, National Professional Development Center on Autism Spectrum Disorders, Frank Porter Graham Child Development Institute.

Kerstein, L. H. (2008). *My sensory book: Working together to explore sensory issues and the big feelings they can cause: A workbook for parents, professionals, and children.* Shawnee Mission: KS: AAPC Publishing.

Lantieri, L. (2008). *Building emotional intelligence: Techniques for cultivating inner strength in children.* Boulder, CO: Sounds True.

Myles, B. S., & Adreon, D. (2001). *Asperger Syndrome and adolescence: Practical solutions for student success.* Shawnee Mission: KS: AAPC Publishing.

van Nieuwenhuijzen, M., Bijman, E. R., Lamberix, I. C., Wijnroks, L., de Castro, B. Orobio, Vermeer, A, & Matthys, W. (2005). Do children do what they say? Responses to hypothetical and real-life social problems in children with mild intellectual disabilities and behavior problems. *Journal of Intellectual Disability Research, 49,* 419-433.

Wilbarger, P., & Wilbarger, J. L. (1991). *Sensory defensiveness in children aged 2-12.* Santa Barbara, CA: Avanti Educational Programs.

Also by Lauren Kerstein ...

My Sensory Book: Working Together to Explore Sensory Issues and the Big Feelings They Can Cause: A Workbook for Parents, Professionals, and Children

My Sensory Book enables children to develop a better understanding of their sensory systems by helping their parents and teachers create an individualized sensory profile. Through numerous strategies broken down by the different sensory systems – tactile, vestibular, proprioception, visual, auditory, gustatory and olfactory – children can learn to cope more effectively with the world around them. This is a practical tool for both home and school.

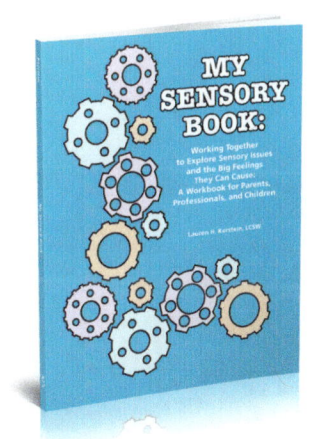

ISBN 9781934575215 | Code 9006 | Price: $22.00

Other Related Books From AAPC ...

Big Picture Thinking: Using Central Coherence Theory to Support Social Skills – A Book for Students

by Aileen Zeitz Collucci, MA, CCC

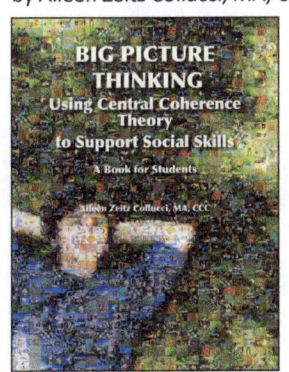

ISBN 9781934575864 | Code 9071 | Price: $25.00

The Incredible 5-Point Scale: The Significantly Improved and Expanded Second Edition; Assisting students in understanding social interactions and controlling their emotional responses

by Kari Dunn Buron and Mitzi Curtis

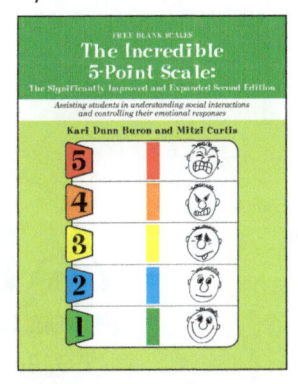

ISBN 9781937473075 | Code 9936A | Price: $20.00

To order, please visit our website at www.aapcpublishing.net

AAPC
PUBLISHING

P.O. Box 23173
Shawnee Mission, Kansas 66283-0173
www.aapcpublishing.net

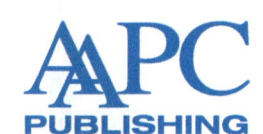

CPSIA information can be obtained at www.ICGtesting.com
Printed in the USA
LVOW01s1915311013

359239LV00004B/7/P